I0702084

Dr. Wilfred Cornelius

PHASES OF FEMALE MIDLIFE

Menopausal Transitions, Post-Menopausal Realities, and Holistic Women's Wellness

Copyright © Wilfred Cornelius 2023. All rights reserved.

No part of this book may be reproduced, distributed, or transmitted in any form or by any means, including photocopying, recording, or other electronic or mechanical methods, without the prior written permission of the author, except in the case of brief quotations embodied in critical reviews and certain other noncommercial uses permitted by copyright law.

ACKNOWLEDGMENT

I am deeply grateful to the many individuals who have contributed to the creation of this book, "Menopause, Post-Menopause, and Women's Health: Exploring the Link to Heart Disease and Osteoporosis." Their unwavering support and invaluable contributions have made this work a reality.

I would like to extend my heartfelt appreciation to the courageous women who shared their stories and experiences of menopause and post-menopause. Your resilience has inspired me to delve deeper into the complexities of women's health and explore the connections to heart disease and osteoporosis.

To my patients, thank you for trusting me with your care and allowing me to be a part of your healthcare journey. Your commitment to well-being has fueled my passion for understanding the intricate links between menopause, heart disease, and osteoporosis.

I am indebted to my esteemed colleagues and fellow oncologists, whose expertise and support have shaped my understanding of women's health. Their guidance and collaboration have been instrumental in expanding my knowledge and enriching the content of this book.

Lastly, I would like to express my profound appreciation to my family, friends, and the readers of this book. Your unwavering support, love, and encouragement have been the driving force behind my efforts. It is my sincere hope that the information and insights shared in this book empower women, inspire medical professionals, and contribute to advancing women's health and well-being.

FOREWORD

In the pages that follow, Dr. Wilfred Cornelius expertly guides us through the intricate terrain of menopause, post-menopause, and the vital connection to heart disease and osteoporosis. As an oncologist with a profound understanding of women's health, he brings to light the often-neglected aspects of this transformative phase in a woman's life. In this thought-provoking book, she unravels the multifaceted relationship between menopause and the two pillars of our well-being: heart health and bone strength.

Throughout history, women have moved mountains, shattered glass ceilings, and carved their own paths against all odds. Yet, amidst their remarkable achievements, their bodies undergo profound transformations that warrant attention, compassion, and understanding. His groundbreaking work serves as a beacon of knowledge, empowering women and healthcare professionals alike to navigate the uncharted waters of menopause with wisdom and grace.

Within these pages, readers will discover a treasure trove of evidence-based insights, comprehensive research, and practical recommendations. Dr. Wilfred Cornelius artfully combines her expertise as an oncologist and her passion for women's health to shed light on the complex interplay between hormonal shifts, heart disease, and osteoporosis. With each turn of the page, a tapestry of understanding is woven, illuminating the path to better health and quality of life for women in the midst of menopause and beyond.

Dr. Wilfred Cornelius's unwavering dedication to her patients and her tireless pursuit of knowledge shines through in this extraordinary book. He expertly dismantles common misconceptions, dispels myths, and invites readers to embrace menopause as a transformative journey — a time of renewal, reinvention, and resilience. Menopause, Post-Menopause, and Women's Health is a testament to the power of knowledge, compassion, and the unwavering spirit of women everywhere.

It is with great pleasure that I invite you to embark upon this enlightening voyage with Dr. Wilfred Cornelius. May this book serve as a trusted companion, empowering you to harness the inherent strength within and embrace the gift of menopause, post-menopause, and all the wonders of women's health.

TABLE OF CONTENT

CHAPTER ONE

Introduction

Contrary to some stereotypes, life doesn't end after menopause. Many women find this stage of life liberating, free from the constraints of monthly periods, and discover new interests and passions.

Menopause is a significant milestone in a woman's life, marking the end of her reproductive years. With this transition comes a myriad of physical, emotional, and hormonal changes that can have a profound impact on her overall health and well-being. As women enter the post-menopausal phase, they face unique challenges and vulnerabilities, particularly when it comes to heart disease and osteoporosis.

In this book, I delve into the intricacies of menopause, post-menopause, heart disease, and osteoporosis. Our aim is to shed light on the connections, uncover the underlying mechanisms, and provide valuable insights for women, healthcare professionals, and researchers alike. Chapter by chapter, we will navigate through the essential aspects of menopause and post-menopause, offering a comprehensive understanding of these life stages. We will explore the hormonal fluctuations that occur during menopause and the subsequent changes in a woman's body and mind. Recognizing the symptoms and emotional impact of menopause is crucial in empowering women to take control of their health during this transformative period.

Heart disease remains a leading cause of death among women worldwide. We will dissect the intricate interplay between menopause and heart health, investigating how hormonal shifts during menopause can influence cardiovascular health and increase the risk of heart disease. By identifying these risk factors and implementing preventive strategies, women can proactively protect their heart health and enjoy a vibrant post-menopausal life. Moreover, we will delve into the silent threat of osteoporosis, a condition characterized by weakened bones and an increased susceptibility to fractures. Exploring the impact of menopause on bone health, we will unravel the hormonal influence on bone loss and discuss methods for early detection, prevention, and treatment of osteoporosis. By addressing this multifaceted issue, we aim to equip women with the knowledge to protect their skeletal integrity and maintain an active, independent lifestyle.

We will also explore the challenges and opportunities of managing heart disease and osteoporosis concurrently during menopause. By adopting a holistic approach that encompasses medical interventions, lifestyle modifications, and self-care practices, women can optimize their health outcomes and maintain a high quality of life. Throughout this book, we emphasize the significance of prioritizing women's health during menopause and post-menopause. Regular health screenings, emotional well-being, and access to supportive networks play vital roles in empowering women to navigate this transformative journey successfully. We also highlight the latest advancements in research, providing insights into potential future directions and innovations in managing menopause-related conditions.

By embarking on this exploration of menopause, post-menopause, heart disease, and osteoporosis, we aspire to empower women to make informed decisions about their health, facilitate proactive healthcare practices, and inspire further research and development in the field. Together, let us embrace the transformative power of knowledge and forge a path towards a healthier, more resilient future for women around the world.

Significance Of Understanding Menopause

Understanding menopause holds immense significance due to its profound impact on a woman's physical, emotional, and mental well-being. This pivotal life stage, marking the cessation of menstrual cycles, necessitates a comprehensive awareness for several reasons.

1. **Health Management:** Awareness of menopause allows women and healthcare professionals to proactively manage health during this transition. Regular check-ups and screenings become crucial in identifying and addressing potential health risks associated with hormonal changes.

2. **Quality of Life:** Menopause brings about a range of symptoms, including hot flashes, mood swings, and sleep disturbances. Understanding these changes enables women to adopt strategies and lifestyle modifications that can enhance their quality of life and alleviate the impact of these symptoms.

3. **Psychological Well-being:** Menopause is not solely a physical process; it significantly influences mental health. Knowledge about the psychological aspects helps women and their support systems to navigate mood fluctuations, anxiety, and potential depressive symptoms, fostering a more resilient mental state.

4. **Informed Decision-Making:** Awareness empowers women to make informed decisions about their health, particularly regarding treatment options such as Hormone Replacement Therapy (HRT).

Informed decision-making, based on a clear understanding of risks and benefits, leads to more personalized and effective healthcare choices.

5. **Relationship Dynamics:** Menopausal symptoms can impact interpersonal relationships. Understanding the emotional and physical changes allows women and their partners to communicate openly, fostering empathy and support during this transitional phase.

6. **Prevention of Health Complications:** Menopause is associated with an increased risk of certain health conditions, including osteoporosis and cardiovascular diseases. Knowledge about these risks enables women to take preventive measures through lifestyle adjustments, regular exercise, and appropriate medical interventions.

7. **Workplace Considerations:** Understanding menopause is essential in the context of the workplace. Awareness facilitates the implementation of supportive policies, accommodations, and a more inclusive work environment, ensuring that women can navigate their professional responsibilities effectively during this phase.

8. **Holistic Approach to Health:** Menopause is a multidimensional experience, and a holistic approach to health becomes paramount. Knowledge about the interconnectedness of

physical, mental, and emotional well-being encourages women to adopt lifestyle changes that encompass nutrition, exercise, stress management, and self-care.

Scope Of The Guide

The scope of this guide on menopause is expansive, aiming to provide a thorough and comprehensive exploration of various facets related to this significant life stage for women. The guide will delve into multiple dimensions, including biological, psychological, and social aspects, to offer a holistic understanding. Here's a detailed note on the scope:

Biological Dimensions:
- **Hormonal Changes:** A detailed examination of the biological underpinnings of menopause, including the hormonal fluctuations and their impact on the female reproductive system.
- **Perimenopause:** In-depth coverage of the transition phase, perimenopause, exploring its duration, early signs, and the physiological changes leading up to menopause.

Symptoms and Challenges:
- **Vasomotor Symptoms:** A comprehensive discussion on the common symptoms experienced

during menopause, such as hot flashes and night sweats.

- **Genitourinary Changes:** Exploration of the impact of hormonal shifts on the urinary and reproductive systems.
- **Cognitive and Emotional Changes:** Examination of the psychological challenges, including mood swings, anxiety, and depression, associated with menopause.

Health Risks and Diagnostics:

- **Cardiovascular and Bone Health:** Thorough coverage of the increased risks of cardiovascular diseases and osteoporosis during and after menopause.
- **Diagnostic Tools:** Explanation of various diagnostic methods, including hormone level testing, bone density scans, and cardiovascular risk assessments.

Management and Treatment Options:

- **Hormone Replacement Therapy (HRT):** Balanced insights into the benefits and risks of HRT, addressing its role in alleviating menopausal symptoms.
- **Lifestyle Modifications:** Detailed guidance on adopting a healthy lifestyle, encompassing nutrition, exercise, and stress management.

Post-Menopause and Ongoing Health:

- **Characteristics of Post-Menopause:** Exploration of the unique aspects of post-menopause, including persistent symptoms and altered health risks.
- **Mental and Emotional Well-being:** Discussion on the importance of ongoing mental health monitoring and strategies for emotional well-being.

Specific Health Dimensions:

- **Bone Health:** Focused content on maintaining bone health through diet, exercise, and potential medical interventions.
- **Cardiovascular Health:** Specialized coverage on cardiovascular health, addressing risks and preventive measures post-menopause.
- **Sexual Health:** In-depth examination of changes in libido and sexual function, along with therapeutic options.

Integrative Approaches and Future Trends:

- **Holistic Healthcare:** Exploration of integrative approaches, including nutrition, supplements, and alternative therapies.
- **Emerging Research Trends:** Insights into the latest advancements in menopausal research, such as personalized medicine and innovative symptom management approaches.

Practical Aspects:

- **Workplace Dynamics:** Examination of the challenges women may face in the workplace during menopause and strategies for support.

Resources for Further Support:

- **Community and Support Groups:** Information on resources, support groups, and online communities to assist women in navigating the challenges of menopause.

CHAPTER TWO

BIOLOGICAL BASIS OF MENOPAUSE

Ovarian Function And Hormonal Changes

Menopause is a natural biological process that marks the end of a woman's reproductive years. It typically occurs in the late 40s or early 50s, and one of the key factors underlying menopause is the decline in ovarian function and the associated hormonal changes. Let's delve into the biological basis of menopause by examining the ovarian function and hormonal changes in detail.

Ovarian Function

The ovaries are the primary reproductive organs in women, responsible for producing eggs (ova) and hormones, including estrogen and progesterone. Ovarian function is tightly regulated by a feedback system involving the hypothalamus, pituitary gland, and ovaries. This system is known as the hypothalamic-pituitary-ovarian (HPO) axis.

1. **Follicular Phase:**

- The menstrual cycle begins with the follicular phase, during which the hypothalamus releases gonadotropin-releasing hormone (GnRH).
- GnRH signals the pituitary gland to release follicle-stimulating hormone (FSH) and luteinizing hormone (LH).
- FSH stimulates the growth of follicles in the ovaries, and each follicle contains an immature egg.

2. **Ovulation:**
- Midway through the menstrual cycle, a surge in LH triggers ovulation, releasing a mature egg from the dominant follicle.

3. **Luteal Phase:**

After ovulation, the ruptured follicle transforms into a structure called the corpus luteum, which produces progesterone.

Progesterone prepares the uterine lining for potential embryo implantation.

Hormonal Changes During Menopause

As women approach menopause, several hormonal changes occur due to the aging of the ovaries. These changes lead to the characteristic symptoms associated with menopause.

1. **Decline in Ovarian Reserve:**
- Ovarian reserve refers to the number and quality of eggs remaining in the ovaries.

- With age, the ovarian reserve decreases, leading to a reduction in the number of follicles and eggs available for ovulation.

2. **Fluctuations in Estrogen Levels:**
- Estrogen, a key hormone produced by the ovaries, begins to decline.
- During the perimenopausal period (the transition to menopause), estrogen levels can fluctuate, leading to irregular menstrual cycles.

3. **Progesterone Decrease:**
- Progesterone production decreases as ovulation becomes irregular.
- This can contribute to changes in the uterine lining and menstrual irregularities.

4. **Menopausal Transition:**
- The period leading up to menopause, known as the menopausal transition, is characterized by hormonal fluctuations and a gradual decline in ovarian function.

5. **Postmenopausal Stage:**
- Menopause is officially declared when a woman has not had a menstrual period for 12 consecutive months.
- After menopause, estrogen and progesterone levels remain low, leading to various postmenopausal symptoms.

Impact of Hormonal Changes

The decline in estrogen and progesterone levels during and after menopause can result in various symptoms, including hot flashes, night sweats, vaginal dryness, mood changes, and bone density loss. Additionally, the decrease in estrogen has broader implications for cardiovascular health and bone health.

Estrogen and Progesterone Levels during Menopause

Menopause, a natural biological process marking the end of a woman's reproductive years, is intricately linked to hormonal changes, particularly in estrogen and progesterone levels. These hormones, produced by the ovaries, play pivotal roles in regulating the menstrual cycle and maintaining reproductive health.

1. **Estrogen Levels**
a. **Pre-Menopausal Dynamics:** In the pre-menopausal phase, the ovaries consistently produce estrogen, a key hormone responsible for the development of female secondary sexual characteristics, regulation of the menstrual cycle, and maintenance of bone density.
b. **Perimenopausal Transition:** As menopause approaches, typically in the late 40s or early 50s,

estrogen levels undergo significant fluctuations during a phase known as perimenopause. This period is characterized by irregular menstrual cycles and varying hormone levels.

c. **Post-Menopausal Decline:** Upon entering menopause, estrogen production significantly decreases. The ovaries produce less estrogen, leading to the cessation of menstruation. Post-menopausal estrogen levels remain consistently lower than during the reproductive years.

d. **Consequences of Estrogen Decline:** The decline in estrogen is associated with various menopausal symptoms, including hot flashes, night sweats, vaginal dryness, and changes in mood. Additionally, lower estrogen levels contribute to long-term health risks such as osteoporosis and cardiovascular disease.

2. Progesterone Levels

a. **Role in the Menstrual Cycle:** Progesterone is another crucial hormone produced by the ovaries. It works in conjunction with estrogen to regulate the menstrual cycle. During the reproductive years, progesterone levels rise after ovulation, preparing the uterus for a potential pregnancy.

b. **Perimenopausal Changes:** Similar to estrogen, progesterone levels fluctuate during perimenopause. As ovulation becomes irregular, there are instances of anovulation (lack of ovulation), leading to variations in progesterone production.

c. **Post-Menopausal Levels:** After menopause, when ovulation ceases, progesterone production declines significantly. Post-menopausal progesterone levels are typically low.

d. **Impact on Symptoms:** While estrogen decline is often associated with vasomotor symptoms, the fluctuations and eventual decline in progesterone can contribute to changes in the menstrual cycle and, in some cases, exacerbate symptoms like mood swings and sleep disturbances.

3. Hormonal Replacement Therapy (HRT)

a. **Addressing Hormonal Imbalance:** Hormone Replacement Therapy (HRT) is a medical intervention that aims to alleviate menopausal symptoms by supplementing estrogen, sometimes in combination with progesterone. This helps balance hormone levels and mitigate associated symptoms.

b. **Considerations and Risks:** However, the use of HRT involves careful consideration of individual health factors and potential risks, such as an increased risk of certain cancers. It should be discussed with healthcare providers to make informed decisions.

Menstrual Irregularities As Precursors To Menopause

Perimenopause, a transitional phase preceding menopause, is characterized by notable hormonal fluctuations, particularly in estrogen and progesterone levels. This phase typically begins in the mid-40s, and its key feature is the variability in menstrual patterns. Menstrual irregularities play a pivotal role in signaling the onset of menopause, providing valuable insights into the biological shifts occurring within a woman's reproductive system

- **Changing Hormone Dynamics:** Hormonal shifts during perimenopause contribute to an environment of imbalance, disrupting the regular hormonal patterns that govern the menstrual cycle. These changes are foundational to understanding the irregularities that manifest during this phase.
- **Variations in Menstrual Cycles:** Menstrual irregularities are evident through deviations in the regularity, duration, and flow of menstrual cycles. Women may experience changes in the length of their menstrual cycles, with intervals between periods becoming irregular and unpredictable.

- **Anovulation and Its Impact:** Anovulation, the absence of ovulation in a menstrual cycle, becomes more prevalent during perimenopause. This phenomenon contributes to the irregularities observed in menstrual cycles, as the usual hormonal cues for ovulation are disrupted.
- **Common Menstrual Patterns:**
1. **Heavy Menstrual Bleeding (Menorrhagia):** The decline in progesterone levels can result in unopposed estrogen effects on the endometrium, leading to heavier menstrual bleeding.
2. **Light or Absent Periods (Oligomenorrhea/Amenorrhea):** Fluctuating hormone levels may cause periods to become lighter or, in some instances, absent altogether.
- **Clinical Indicators and Assessments:** Healthcare professionals employ specific markers to assess perimenopause:
1. **Follicle-Stimulating Hormone (FSH) Levels:** Elevated FSH levels signify reduced ovarian responsiveness and are indicative of perimenopause.
2. **Anti-Mullerian Hormone (AMH) Levels:** Decreasing AMH levels reflect a diminished ovarian reserve and are associated with irregular menstrual patterns.
- **Significance for Women and Healthcare Providers:** Recognizing menstrual irregularities as precursors

to menopause holds crucial importance for women navigating this transitional phase. It serves as a biological roadmap, offering insights into fertility considerations, family planning, and the potential onset of menopausal symptoms.

- **Monitoring and Support:** Regular monitoring of menstrual patterns, coupled with hormonal assessments, empowers women and healthcare providers to proactively manage the challenges associated with perimenopause. This approach facilitates informed decision-making and ensures comprehensive support throughout this transformative journey.

CHAPTER THREE

PERIMENOPAUSE: THE TRANSITION PHASE

Definition and Duration

Perimenopause, often referred to as the menopausal transition, signifies a natural and intricate phase in a woman's reproductive life. It is characterized by the gradual onset of hormonal changes that precede menopause, marking the end of the childbearing years.

The duration of perimenopause is a variable and individualized aspect of this transitional phase. Typically commencing in the mid-40s, the onset may vary among women. The entire perimenopausal journey spans several years, extending from a few months to up to a decade before the actual onset of menopause.

Central to perimenopause are significant shifts in hormonal levels, particularly estrogen and progesterone. These fluctuations instigate a series of changes within the reproductive system, contributing to irregularities in the menstrual cycle. A distinguishing feature of perimenopause is the increased variability in ovulation. Women may experience cycles where ovulation does not occur, leading to inconsistent menstrual patterns. This irregularity serves as a significant indicator of the commencement of the menopausal transition.

Menstrual Irregularities:

Irregularities in menstrual cycles become a hallmark of perimenopause. Changes in the length of menstrual cycles and irregular intervals between periods are common occurrences. These variations underscore the dynamic nature of the transition.

Physical and Psychological Symptoms:

Perimenopause is associated with a spectrum of physical and psychological symptoms. Hot flashes, night sweats, mood swings, and alterations in sleep patterns are prevalent during this phase. The intensity and duration of these symptoms can vary widely among women.

Fertility Considerations:

While fertility declines during perimenopause, conception remains possible. However, the unpredictable ovulation patterns and hormonal changes introduce challenges associated with family planning during this transitional period.

Individual Variability:
Recognizing the individual variability in the experience of perimenopause is paramount. Genetic factors, overall health, and lifestyle choices contribute to the diverse manifestations of symptoms, emphasizing the personalized nature of this life stage.

Medical Guidance and Support:
Given the dynamic nature of perimenopause, seeking medical guidance is crucial. Healthcare providers play a vital role in offering support, monitoring hormonal changes, and providing interventions to manage symptoms effectively.

Empowerment Through Understanding:
Understanding the definition and duration of perimenopause empowers women to navigate this transitional phase with knowledge and preparedness. It fosters open communication with healthcare providers and facilitates informed decision-making regarding family planning and effective management of menopausal symptoms.

Early Signs And Symptoms

As women navigate the complex terrain of perimenopause, various early signs and symptoms emerge, serving as harbingers of the impending transition. Recognizing these indicators is pivotal for women and healthcare providers alike in understanding and managing the transformative journey through perimenopause.

1. **Irregular Menstrual Cycles:** One of the earliest and most prominent signs of perimenopause is irregularities in menstrual cycles. Women may experience variations in the length of their menstrual cycles, with intervals between periods becoming irregular. This irregularity stems from hormonal fluctuations affecting ovulation.

2. **Changes in Menstrual Flow:** Alongside irregular cycles, perimenopausal women often observe alterations in menstrual flow. This may manifest as changes in the volume and duration of menstrual bleeding, ranging from heavier flows to lighter periods.

3. **Hot Flashes and Night Sweats:** Hot flashes, characterized by sudden sensations of heat, and night sweats are common early symptoms of perimenopause. These episodic temperature fluctuations can disrupt sleep patterns and significantly impact a woman's daily life.

4. **Mood Swings and Emotional Changes:** Hormonal shifts during perimenopause can influence mood and emotions. Women may experience mood swings, irritability, and heightened emotional

sensitivity. Anxiety and depression can also surface during this phase.

5. **Sleep Disturbances:** Changes in sleep patterns often accompany perimenopause. Women may find it challenging to fall asleep or stay asleep, leading to fatigue and daytime sleepiness. Night sweats can contribute to sleep disturbances as well.

6. **Vaginal Dryness and Discomfort:** Hormonal changes can affect the moisture and elasticity of vaginal tissues, resulting in vaginal dryness and discomfort. This can lead to pain during intercourse and increased susceptibility to urinary tract infections.

7. **Changes in Libido:** Fluctuations in hormone levels may influence a woman's sexual desire and arousal. Some women may experience a decrease in libido during perimenopause, while others may notice an increase.

8. **Breast Tenderness:** Breast tenderness and changes in breast tissue are early physical manifestations of perimenopause. Hormonal fluctuations can lead to increased sensitivity and discomfort in the breast area.

9. **Weight Gain and Metabolic Changes:** Metabolic changes, including a decrease in metabolic rate, can contribute to weight gain during perimenopause. Changes in body composition,

particularly an increase in abdominal fat, are common.

10. **Headaches and Migraines:** Some women may experience an increase in the frequency and intensity of headaches or migraines during perimenopause. Hormonal fluctuations are believed to play a role in triggering these symptoms.

11. **Joint Pain and Muscle Aches:** Hormonal changes can affect connective tissues, leading to joint pain and muscle aches. Some women may notice increased stiffness and discomfort, particularly in the morning.

12. **Memory and Cognitive Changes:** Cognitive changes, including lapses in memory and difficulty concentrating, may manifest during perimenopause. These changes are often attributed to hormonal fluctuations affecting brain function

Hormonal Fluctuations

Hormonal fluctuations are at the heart of perimenopause, driving the physiological changes that characterize this transitional phase in a woman's life. Understanding the intricacies of these hormonal shifts is essential for women and healthcare providers alike, as they play a central role in the diverse array of symptoms experienced during perimenopause.

1. **Estrogen Variations:** One of the primary hormonal players in perimenopause is estrogen. During this transitional phase, estrogen levels exhibit fluctuations, often marked by an overall decline. This hormonal variability is a key factor influencing the various symptoms associated with perimenopause.
2. **Progesterone Fluctuations:** Progesterone, another crucial reproductive hormone, also undergoes fluctuations during perimenopause. The balance between estrogen and progesterone is disrupted, contributing to irregularities in the menstrual cycle and affecting the overall hormonal milieu.
3. **Ovarian Function Changes:** Perimenopause is characterized by changes in ovarian function. The ovaries, which are responsible for producing and releasing eggs, experience a decline in their reproductive capacity. This decline is associated with a decrease in the production of estrogen and progesterone.
4. **Anovulation:** Anovulation, the absence of ovulation in a menstrual cycle, becomes more prevalent during perimenopause. This results in hormonal imbalances, contributing to irregular menstrual cycles and variations in the quality of the endometrial lining.
5. **Follicle-Stimulating Hormone (FSH) Levels:** As ovarian function declines, the pituitary gland

releases higher levels of follicle-stimulating hormone (FSH) in an attempt to stimulate ovulation. Elevated FSH levels are a hallmark of perimenopause and are often used as a diagnostic marker.

6. **Luteinizing Hormone (LH) Fluctuations:** Luteinizing hormone (LH), which works in conjunction with FSH to regulate the menstrual cycle, also undergoes fluctuations. The increased levels of LH, particularly in relation to FSH, contribute to the overall hormonal imbalance observed in perimenopause.

7. **Impact on the Hypothalamus-Pituitary-Ovarian Axis:** The intricate interplay between the hypothalamus, pituitary gland, and ovaries, known as the hypothalamus-pituitary-ovarian (HPO) axis, is disrupted during perimenopause. This disruption leads to dysregulation in the production and secretion of reproductive hormones.

8. **Estrogen Dominance and Relative Progesterone Deficiency:** As ovarian function declines, there is a tendency towards estrogen dominance due to a relative deficiency in progesterone. This imbalance contributes to changes in the endometrial lining and can lead to conditions such as heavy menstrual bleeding.

9. **Impact on Mood and Emotional Well-being:** Hormonal fluctuations in perimenopause can have a profound impact on mood and emotional well-being. Estrogen, in particular, influences neurotransmitters like serotonin and norepinephrine, contributing to mood swings, irritability, and heightened emotional sensitivity.

10. **Vasomotor Symptoms:** Fluctuations in estrogen levels are closely linked to vasomotor symptoms, including hot flashes and night sweats. The mechanism behind these symptoms is not fully understood, but it is believed to involve the hypothalamus, which regulates body temperature.

11. **Bone Health Implications:** Estrogen plays a crucial role in maintaining bone density. The decline in estrogen levels during perimenopause contributes to an increased risk of osteoporosis and bone fractures.

Impact On Menstrual Cycles

The transition through perimenopause brings about a multitude of changes in a woman's menstrual cycles, reflecting the complex interplay of hormonal fluctuations. These alterations in the regularity, duration, and characteristics of menstrual cycles are pivotal aspects of perimenopause and contribute significantly to the overall experience of this life stage.

1. **Irregular Menstrual Cycles:** One of the hallmark impacts of perimenopause on menstrual cycles is irregularity. Women may notice variations in the length of their menstrual cycles, with intervals between periods becoming unpredictable. This irregularity stems from the hormonal fluctuations, particularly the decline in estrogen and progesterone.

2. **Anovulation:** Anovulation, the absence of ovulation in a menstrual cycle, becomes more prevalent during perimenopause. This contributes to irregular cycles as the typical hormonal patterns regulating the menstrual cycle are disrupted. Anovulation is a key factor in the variability observed in perimenopausal menstrual patterns.

3. **Changes in Menstrual Flow:** Alongside irregular cycles, perimenopausal women often experience changes in menstrual flow. Fluctuations in hormonal levels, particularly a relative excess of estrogen compared to progesterone, can lead to alterations in the volume and duration of menstrual bleeding. This may manifest as heavier or lighter periods.

4. **Heavy Menstrual Bleeding (Menorrhagia):** Declining progesterone levels and an imbalance with estrogen can result in unopposed estrogen effects on the endometrium. This can lead to heavy menstrual bleeding, known as menorrhagia.

Menorrhagia is a common manifestation of perimenopausal hormonal changes and can impact a woman's quality of life.

5. **Light or Absent Periods (Oligomenorrhea/Amenorrhea):** On the other end of the spectrum, some women may experience lighter periods or, in some instances, periods that become increasingly sparse. Oligomenorrhea refers to infrequent menstruation, while amenorrhea denotes the absence of menstruation for several cycles.

6. **Variable Menstrual Symptoms:** The variability in hormonal levels can influence the spectrum of menstrual symptoms experienced by women during perimenopause. Some may notice an exacerbation of premenstrual symptoms, while others may find relief from symptoms they previously experienced.

7. **Impact on Fertility:** While fertility declines during perimenopause, the irregularity in menstrual cycles can pose challenges for women attempting conception. The unpredictable ovulation patterns make it more difficult to time intercourse for optimal fertility.

8. **Diagnostic Value:** The changes in menstrual cycles serve as diagnostic indicators of perimenopause. Elevated levels of follicle-stimulating hormone (FSH) and irregular cycles are often used by

healthcare providers to confirm the onset of perimenopause.

9. **Emotional and Practical Implications:** The impact on menstrual cycles goes beyond the physical realm, extending to emotional and practical considerations. Women may find it challenging to predict and plan for their periods, leading to a need for increased preparedness and adaptability.

CHAPTER FOUR

COMMON SYMPTOMS AND CHALLENGES

Vasomotor Symptoms

Vasomotor symptoms represent a prominent and often challenging aspect of perimenopause, encompassing a range of physiological experiences that profoundly impact a woman's quality of life. These symptoms, primarily driven by hormonal fluctuations, can manifest in various ways, with hot flashes and night sweats being the most prevalent. This detailed note aims to comprehensively explore vasomotor symptoms, shedding light on their nature, underlying mechanisms, and the challenges they pose during the perimenopausal transition.

1. **Hot Flashes:** Hot flashes are sudden, intense sensations of heat that typically originate in the upper body and radiate upwards. These episodes can last for a few seconds to several minutes, causing flushing, sweating, and an overall feeling of warmth.

2. **Night Sweats:** Night sweats are nocturnal manifestations of hot flashes, disrupting sleep patterns and contributing to sleep disturbances

during perimenopause. The sudden onset of intense sweating during sleep can lead to discomfort and repeated awakenings.

3. **Frequency and Duration:** Vasomotor symptoms, especially hot flashes, vary widely in terms of frequency and duration. Some women may experience occasional, mild episodes, while others may endure frequent and severe occurrences. The duration of these symptoms can extend for several years during perimenopause.

4. **Hormonal Mechanisms:** The precise mechanisms behind vasomotor symptoms are linked to hormonal fluctuations, particularly the decline in estrogen levels. Estrogen plays a role in regulating the body's internal thermostat, and its reduced levels during perimenopause contribute to the dysregulation of temperature control.

5. **Impact on Quality of Life:** Vasomotor symptoms can have a profound impact on a woman's overall quality of life. The unpredictability and intensity of hot flashes, especially when coupled with night sweats, can lead to chronic fatigue, irritability, and mood disturbances.

6. **Sleep Disturbances:** Night sweats, in particular, contribute to sleep disturbances and insomnia during perimenopause. The disruption of sleep patterns can lead to daytime fatigue, impaired

concentration, and an overall decline in mental well-being.

7. **Emotional and Psychological Impact:** The psychological impact of vasomotor symptoms should not be underestimated. Women may experience heightened anxiety, frustration, and a sense of loss of control over their bodies. These emotional challenges add an additional layer of complexity to the perimenopausal experience.

8. **Triggers and Aggravating Factors:** Certain triggers and aggravating factors can exacerbate vasomotor symptoms. These include stress, caffeine, spicy foods, alcohol, and exposure to hot environments. Identifying and managing these factors can contribute to symptom alleviation.

9. **Management Strategies:** Various management strategies exist to alleviate vasomotor symptoms. Hormone Replacement Therapy (HRT), lifestyle modifications, cognitive-behavioral therapy, and herbal supplements are among the approaches employed to mitigate the impact of hot flashes and night sweats.

10. **Individual Variability:** It's crucial to recognize the individual variability in the experience of vasomotor symptoms. While some women may navigate perimenopause with minimal disruption, others may find these symptoms significantly

challenging. Factors such as genetics, overall health, and lifestyle contribute to this diversity.

11. **Long-term Health Considerations:** Emerging research suggests that the experience of vasomotor symptoms during perimenopause may have implications for long-term health. Understanding the potential links between these symptoms and cardiovascular health, bone density, and cognitive function is an active area of investigation.

Genitourinary Changes

As women transition through perimenopause, a phase marked by hormonal fluctuations and reproductive changes, they often encounter significant alterations in the genitourinary system. These changes can impact various aspects of urogenital health, giving rise to common symptoms and challenges that warrant attention and understanding.

1. **Vaginal Dryness:** A prevalent genitourinary change during perimenopause is vaginal dryness. Declining estrogen levels contribute to a reduction in vaginal lubrication, leading to dryness and discomfort. This can result in pain or irritation during sexual activity and an increased susceptibility to vaginal infections.

2. **Vaginal Atrophy:** Estrogen plays a vital role in maintaining the health and elasticity of vaginal

tissues. Reduced estrogen levels during perimenopause can lead to vaginal atrophy, characterized by thinning, inflammation, and a loss of lubrication. Vaginal atrophy contributes to discomfort, pain, and may impact sexual function.

3. **Dyspareunia:** Dyspareunia, or painful intercourse, is a common symptom associated with genitourinary changes in perimenopause. Vaginal dryness and atrophy can make sexual activity uncomfortable, affecting the quality of a woman's intimate relationships.

4. **Urinary Incontinence:** Changes in pelvic floor muscles and connective tissues, influenced by hormonal fluctuations, can contribute to urinary incontinence. Women may experience stress incontinence, where activities like laughing, coughing, or sneezing lead to unintentional urine leakage.

5. **Increased UTI Risk:** Reduced vaginal acidity and changes in the microbiome increase the risk of urinary tract infections (UTIs). The genitourinary changes in perimenopause create an environment conducive to bacterial growth, potentially causing recurrent UTIs.

6. **Frequency and Urgency of Urination:** Hormonal shifts can affect the bladder and urethra, leading to an increased frequency of urination and a sense of urgency. Women may find themselves needing to

urinate more frequently, especially during the night, impacting sleep patterns.

7. **Pelvic Organ Prolapse:** Weakening of pelvic floor muscles can contribute to pelvic organ prolapse, where pelvic organs, such as the bladder or uterus, descend into the vaginal space. This can lead to sensations of pressure or fullness in the pelvic region.

8. **Changes in Libido:** Genitourinary changes, including vaginal dryness and discomfort, can influence sexual desire and arousal. These changes may contribute to a decline in libido, impacting a woman's overall sexual well-being.

9. **Impact on Emotional Well-being:** The genitourinary symptoms and challenges in perimenopause can have emotional implications. Women may experience feelings of frustration, embarrassment, or a sense of loss regarding their sexual health. Open communication with healthcare providers and partners is essential for addressing emotional concerns.

10. **Preventive and Therapeutic Approaches:** Various preventive and therapeutic approaches can address genitourinary changes during perimenopause. Hormone replacement therapy (HRT) and local estrogen therapies, such as vaginal estrogen creams, can be effective in managing symptoms. Pelvic floor exercises and

lifestyle modifications also play a crucial role in improving urogenital health.

Sleep Disturbances

Perimenopause, the transitional phase leading to menopause, is often accompanied by significant changes in sleep patterns. These disturbances can have profound effects on a woman's overall well-being, impacting her physical health, emotional resilience, and daily functioning. Understanding the nature of sleep disturbances during perimenopause is essential for implementing effective strategies to improve sleep quality and mitigate associated challenges.

1. **Insomnia:** Insomnia, characterized by difficulty falling asleep, staying asleep, or experiencing non-restorative sleep, is a common sleep disturbance during perimenopause. Hormonal fluctuations, particularly changes in estrogen and progesterone, can contribute to the onset of insomnia.

2. **Night Sweats:** Night sweats, episodes of excessive sweating during sleep, are a vasomotor symptom associated with hormonal changes in perimenopause. These can lead to disrupted sleep, causing women to wake up multiple times during the night, impacting sleep continuity.

3. **Hot Flashes:** Hot flashes, sudden sensations of heat typically accompanied by flushing and sweating, are prevalent during perimenopause. These can occur both during the day and at night, contributing to sleep interruptions and overall discomfort.

4. **Changes in Sleep Architecture:** Hormonal fluctuations influence sleep architecture, altering the proportion of time spent in different sleep stages. Perimenopausal women may experience changes in the duration of rapid eye movement (REM) sleep and deep sleep, affecting the overall quality of sleep.

5. **Sleep Fragmentation:** Nighttime awakenings and interruptions, often linked to hormonal fluctuations and vasomotor symptoms, contribute to sleep fragmentation. Women may find it challenging to achieve continuous, restorative sleep, leading to feelings of fatigue and daytime sleepiness.

6. **Increased Sensitivity to Environmental Factors:** Hormonal changes during perimenopause can heighten sensitivity to environmental factors that impact sleep, such as temperature, noise, and light. Women may find themselves more affected by these external factors, further contributing to sleep disturbances.

7. **Anxiety and Stress:** The emotional challenges associated with perimenopause, including mood swings and increased stress, can exacerbate sleep disturbances. Anxiety about hormonal changes, aging, and other life transitions may contribute to difficulty relaxing and falling asleep.
8. **Cognitive Impact:** Sleep disturbances in perimenopause can have cognitive repercussions, affecting memory, concentration, and overall cognitive function. Persistent sleep difficulties may contribute to feelings of cognitive fogginess and reduced daytime alertness.
9. **Impact on Mood and Emotional Well-being:** Sleep disturbances can influence mood and emotional well-being. Chronic sleep disruptions are associated with an increased risk of mood disorders, including depression and irritability. Addressing sleep issues is crucial for supporting emotional resilience during perimenopause.
10. **Comprehensive Sleep Management:** Managing sleep disturbances during perimenopause involves a comprehensive approach. Lifestyle modifications, such as maintaining a consistent sleep schedule, creating a conducive sleep environment, and engaging in relaxation techniques, can contribute to better sleep hygiene.
11. **Medical Interventions:** In some cases, medical interventions, including hormone replacement

therapy (HRT) or other medications, may be recommended to address severe sleep disturbances. Consultation with a healthcare provider is essential to determine the most appropriate intervention based on individual health considerations.

Cognitive Changes

Perimenopause is associated with various cognitive changes that can impact memory, concentration, and overall cognitive function. While cognitive changes during perimenopause are a natural part of the aging process, hormonal fluctuations play a significant role in shaping the nature and extent of these changes. Understanding the cognitive landscape of perimenopause is crucial for women and healthcare providers to navigate this phase with awareness and proactive management.

1. **Memory Changes:** Memory changes are a common cognitive aspect affected during perimenopause. Women may notice lapses in memory, including forgetfulness, difficulty recalling names or details, and occasional "brain fog." Hormonal fluctuations, particularly changes in estrogen levels, are implicated in these memory changes.

2. **Impact on Short-Term Memory:** Short-term memory, responsible for holding and processing

information for brief periods, may be particularly affected. Women in perimenopause might find it challenging to retain and recall recently learned information, contributing to the perception of memory difficulties.

3. **Attention and Concentration:** Cognitive changes during perimenopause can influence attention and concentration. Women may experience difficulty maintaining focus on tasks, increased distractibility, and a reduced ability to concentrate for extended periods. These changes can impact daily productivity and task performance.

4. **Word Retrieval Difficulty:** Some women may experience difficulty with word retrieval, often referred to as the "tip-of-the-tongue" phenomenon. This involves temporarily struggling to recall specific words or names, a phenomenon influenced by cognitive processes linked to language and memory.

5. **Executive Function Changes:** Executive functions, encompassing skills like planning, organizing, and problem-solving, may be subtly affected during perimenopause. Women may find it challenging to manage multiple tasks simultaneously or initiate and complete complex cognitive activities.

6. **Mood and Cognitive Interaction:** The interplay between mood changes and cognitive function is noteworthy during perimenopause. Mood swings,

anxiety, or irritability can influence cognitive performance, creating a complex relationship between emotional well-being and cognitive function.

7. **Hormonal Influence on Cognitive Changes:** Hormones, especially estrogen, play a crucial role in maintaining cognitive function. Estrogen receptors are present in various areas of the brain associated with memory and cognitive processes. Fluctuations in estrogen levels during perimenopause contribute to changes in these cognitive functions.

8. **Sleep Disturbances and Cognitive Impact:** Sleep disturbances, common during perimenopause, can contribute to cognitive changes. Disrupted sleep patterns, including insomnia and night sweats, can lead to fatigue and reduced cognitive alertness, impacting memory consolidation and overall cognitive performance.

9. **Individual Variability:** It is essential to recognize the individual variability in the experience of cognitive changes during perimenopause. Some women may navigate this phase with minimal cognitive impact, while others may find certain aspects more challenging. Factors such as genetics, lifestyle, and overall health contribute to this diversity.

10. **Coping Strategies and Cognitive Health:** Implementing effective coping strategies can support cognitive health during perimenopause. These strategies include maintaining a healthy lifestyle with regular exercise, a balanced diet, stress management, and engaging in activities that stimulate cognitive function, such as puzzles and mental exercises.

11. **Seeking Professional Guidance:** Women experiencing significant cognitive changes or concerns should seek professional guidance. A healthcare provider can conduct assessments to evaluate cognitive function, rule out other potential causes, and offer recommendations or interventions if necessary.

Emotional And Psychological Impact

Perimenopause is characterized not only by physical changes but also by a range of emotional and psychological impacts. The interplay of hormonal fluctuations, life stage transitions, and individual variability contributes to a complex landscape of emotional experiences during perimenopause. Understanding and addressing these emotional and psychological aspects are vital for promoting mental well-being and resilience during this transformative phase.

1. **Mood Swings:** Hormonal fluctuations, particularly changes in estrogen and progesterone levels, can contribute to mood swings. Women may experience sudden shifts in mood, ranging from elation to irritability or sadness. These mood swings are often linked to the dynamic hormonal changes inherent in perimenopause.
2. **Increased Vulnerability to Stress:** Perimenopause can amplify stress sensitivity. Women may find themselves more susceptible to stressors, both related to menopausal changes and external life factors. Elevated stress levels can contribute to emotional reactivity and a heightened sense of overwhelm.
3. **Anxiety and Worry:** Anxiety, characterized by excessive worry and apprehension, can manifest or intensify during perimenopause. Concerns about aging, hormonal changes, and the uncertainty of this life stage may contribute to heightened anxiety levels.
4. **Depressive Symptoms:** Some women may experience symptoms of depression during perimenopause. Changes in hormone levels, coupled with life transitions and societal expectations, can contribute to feelings of sadness, hopelessness, and a diminished interest in previously enjoyed activities.

5. **Irritability and Tension:** Hormonal fluctuations can contribute to increased irritability and tension. Women may find themselves more reactive to daily stressors, and interpersonal relationships may be affected by heightened emotional responses.

6. **Changes in Self-Identity:** Perimenopause often coincides with significant life changes, including potential shifts in roles and identity. Women may grapple with questions of self-worth, body image, and societal expectations, contributing to emotional introspection and self-reflection.

7. **Impact on Relationships:** Emotional changes during perimenopause can influence relationships. Communication patterns, intimacy, and overall relationship dynamics may be affected. Open communication with partners and loved ones is crucial for navigating these changes collaboratively.

8. **Sleep Disturbances and Emotional Well-being:** Sleep disturbances, common during perimenopause, can impact emotional well-being. Fatigue and disrupted sleep patterns can exacerbate mood swings, irritability, and stress sensitivity, creating a cyclical relationship between sleep and emotional health.

9. **Coping Mechanisms and Adaptation:** Adopting effective coping mechanisms is essential for

managing emotional challenges during perimenopause. Mindfulness practices, relaxation techniques, regular exercise, and seeking social support can contribute to emotional resilience and adaptation.

10. **Emotional Intelligence:** Cultivating emotional intelligence, which involves recognizing, understanding, and managing one's own emotions, becomes particularly valuable during perimenopause. Developing emotional awareness allows women to navigate emotional changes with greater self-compassion and understanding.

11. **Professional Support:** Seeking professional support, such as counseling or therapy, can provide a safe space to explore and address emotional concerns. Mental health professionals can offer guidance, coping strategies, and a supportive environment for women experiencing significant emotional challenges.

12. **Empowerment Through Education:** Education and awareness about the emotional and psychological aspects of perimenopause empower women to approach this life stage with knowledge and preparedness. Understanding that emotional changes are a normal part of the menopausal transition fosters a proactive mindset.

CHAPTER FIVE

HEALTH RISKS DURING MENOPAUSE

Cardiovascular Health

Menopause brings about hormonal changes that can influence various aspects of health, including cardiovascular health. Understanding the intricate connections between menopause and cardiovascular well-being is crucial for women and healthcare providers alike. Here's a comprehensive examination of the impact of menopause on cardiovascular health and strategies for maintaining a heart-healthy lifestyle:

Hormonal Changes and Cardiovascular Impact:
Menopause is characterized by a decline in estrogen levels. Estrogen, known for its protective effects on the cardiovascular system, plays a role in maintaining healthy blood vessels, regulating cholesterol levels, and promoting overall cardiovascular function. The decrease in estrogen during menopause can contribute to changes in the cardiovascular landscape.

Cardiovascular Risk Factors:

Menopause can influence several cardiovascular risk factors:

1. **Changes in Lipid Profile:** Estrogen helps regulate cholesterol levels. With its decline, there may be an increase in low-density lipoprotein (LDL) cholesterol and a decrease in high-density lipoprotein (HDL) cholesterol.
2. **Blood Pressure Fluctuations:** Blood pressure may fluctuate during menopause, and some women may experience increases in blood pressure levels.
3. **Weight Redistribution:** Changes in hormonal balance can contribute to a redistribution of body fat, with an increased tendency for abdominal or visceral fat accumulation, which is associated with cardiovascular risk.

Increased Cardiovascular Disease (CVD) Risk:

The postmenopausal period is associated with an increased risk of cardiovascular diseases (CVD). Women, particularly those without previous cardiovascular concerns, may see a convergence of risk factors leading to an elevated likelihood of heart disease.

Vascular Changes:

Estrogen withdrawal during menopause can lead to changes in the structure and function of blood vessels. Arterial stiffness may increase, potentially contributing to elevated blood pressure and reduced cardiovascular efficiency.

Impact on Endothelial Function:
Estrogen has a protective effect on the endothelium, the inner lining of blood vessels. Its decline during menopause may impair endothelial function, affecting the regulation of blood flow and vascular tone.

Menopausal Symptoms and Cardiovascular Correlation:
Certain menopausal symptoms, such as hot flashes and night sweats, may be linked to cardiovascular changes. Emerging research suggests that women experiencing more severe menopausal symptoms may have a higher risk of cardiovascular events.

Lifestyle Factors and Cardiovascular Health:
Adopting a heart-healthy lifestyle is crucial during menopause and beyond:
1. **Regular Physical Activity:** Exercise helps maintain cardiovascular fitness, manage weight, and regulate blood pressure. Both aerobic and strength-training exercises are beneficial.
2. **Healthy Diet:** Emphasizing a diet rich in fruits, vegetables, whole grains, and lean proteins contributes to optimal cardiovascular health.

Limiting saturated fats, cholesterol, and processed foods is essential.

3. **Smoking Cessation:** Quitting smoking is paramount for cardiovascular health. Smoking is a significant risk factor for heart disease.

4. **Moderate Alcohol Consumption:** If alcohol is consumed, it should be in moderation. Excessive alcohol intake can contribute to cardiovascular risk.

Bone Health Medications and Cardiovascular Considerations:

Some medications prescribed for bone health, such as bisphosphonates, may have potential cardiovascular benefits. However, individual considerations and discussions with healthcare providers are essential.

Hormone Replacement Therapy (HRT) and Cardiovascular Risk:

The use of hormone replacement therapy (HRT) during menopause is a complex consideration. While it may alleviate menopausal symptoms, its impact on cardiovascular health is subject to ongoing research and should be discussed with healthcare providers, weighing potential risks and benefits.

Regular Cardiovascular Assessments:

Regular cardiovascular assessments, including blood pressure monitoring, cholesterol screenings, and assessments of other risk factors, are essential during and after menopause. These assessments aid in the early detection and management of cardiovascular issues.

Mental Health and Cardiovascular Impact:
The psychological impact of menopause, including stress and mood changes, can influence cardiovascular health. Strategies for managing stress and prioritizing mental health contribute to overall cardiovascular well-being.

Multidisciplinary Approach to Care:
A multidisciplinary approach involving healthcare providers, including gynecologists, cardiologists, and lifestyle specialists, is crucial for comprehensive cardiovascular care during menopause. Individualized care plans address unique health needs.

Bone Health and Osteoporosis

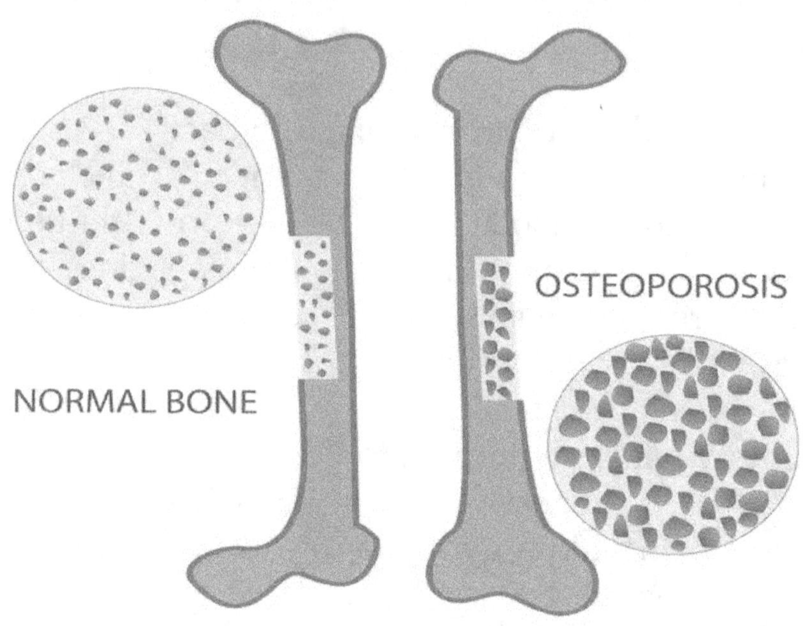

Menstruation is marked by hormonal changes that have far-reaching effects, including impacts on bone health. The decline in estrogen levels during menopause becomes a pivotal factor influencing bone density, placing women at an increased risk of osteoporosis. Understanding the intricacies of this relationship is essential for women and healthcare providers to implement proactive strategies, ensuring optimal bone health during and after menopause.

1. **Estrogen's Role in Bone Health:** Estrogen plays a crucial role in maintaining bone density by supporting the balance between bone formation and resorption. As menopause progresses, the decline in estrogen levels disrupts this equilibrium, leading to an increased rate of bone loss.

2. **Accelerated Bone Loss:** In the initial years of menopause, women may experience accelerated bone loss, particularly in trabecular bone (spongy bone tissue). This loss contributes to an increased susceptibility to fractures and a reduction in overall bone density.

3. **Osteoporosis Risk:** The cumulative effect of hormonal changes and accelerated bone loss places menopausal women at a heightened risk of developing osteoporosis. Osteoporosis is a condition characterized by porous and brittle bones, significantly increasing the likelihood of fractures, particularly in areas such as the spine, hips, and wrists.

4. **Vertebral Fractures:** Osteoporosis-related vertebral fractures are common among menopausal women. These fractures can lead to changes in posture, height reduction, and chronic pain. The vertebral fractures may occur with minimal trauma or even spontaneously.

5. **Hip Fractures:** The risk of hip fractures rises significantly during menopause due to decreased

bone density. Hip fractures are associated with substantial morbidity and mortality, making prevention a critical aspect of managing bone health in menopausal women.

6. **Impact on Quality of Life:** Osteoporosis-related fractures can have a profound impact on the quality of life for menopausal women. Functional limitations, increased dependency, and the emotional toll of fractures contribute to a complex interplay of physical and psychological challenges.

7. **Lifestyle Factors:** Lifestyle factors play a crucial role in bone health during menopause. Adequate intake of calcium and vitamin D, regular weight-bearing exercises, and a healthy lifestyle contribute to maintaining bone density and mitigating the risk of osteoporosis.

8. **Bone Mineral Density (BMD) Testing:** Bone mineral density (BMD) testing is a valuable tool for assessing bone health in menopausal women. This non-invasive test provides insights into bone density levels, guiding healthcare providers in determining the need for preventive measures or interventions.

9. **Hormone Replacement Therapy (HRT):** Hormone replacement therapy (HRT) may be considered for some menopausal women to address hormonal deficiencies. Estrogen replacement can help mitigate bone loss; however, the decision to

undergo HRT should be individualized, considering potential risks and benefits.

- **Calcium and Vitamin D Supplementation:** Adequate calcium and vitamin D intake are essential for maintaining bone health. Menopausal women may require supplementation if dietary sources are insufficient. Healthcare providers can guide women in determining appropriate supplementation based on individual needs.
- **Exercise and Physical Activity:** Weight-bearing exercises, such as walking, jogging, and resistance training, contribute to bone health by stimulating bone formation. Incorporating regular physical activity into a routine is beneficial for overall bone density and strength.
- **Smoking and Alcohol:** Smoking and excessive alcohol consumption are detrimental to bone health. Menopausal women are advised to avoid smoking and limit alcohol intake to support optimal bone density and reduce the risk of fractures.
- **Multidisciplinary Approach:** Managing bone health during and after menopause requires a multidisciplinary approach. Collaboration between gynecologists, endocrinologists, nutritionists, and physical therapists ensures a comprehensive

strategy tailored to the individual needs of each woman.

- **Patient Education and Empowerment:** Educating menopausal women about the importance of bone health and osteoporosis prevention empowers them to take an active role in their well-being. Understanding risk factors, lifestyle modifications, and available interventions enhances informed decision-making.

Weight Gain and Metabolic Changes

Menopause, a natural and inevitable phase in a woman's life, is accompanied by a myriad of hormonal shifts that influence various aspects of health, including metabolism and body weight. Understanding the intricate relationship between menopause, weight gain, and metabolic changes is essential for women and healthcare providers alike. This comprehensive exploration delves into the physiological factors, lifestyle influences, and preventive strategies associated with weight gain and metabolic alterations during and after menopause.

1. **Hormonal Dynamics:** Menopause is characterized by a decline in estrogen and progesterone levels. These hormonal changes can contribute to shifts in body composition, including an increase in visceral fat. Estrogen, in particular, plays a role in

regulating body weight and metabolism, and its reduction during menopause can influence weight distribution.

2. **Changes in Body Composition:** Menopausal women often experience changes in body composition, with a tendency to gain fat, especially around the abdomen. This shift is linked to hormonal fluctuations, aging, and a decrease in lean muscle mass, collectively contributing to alterations in metabolic function.

3. **Metabolic Rate Decline:** With aging and hormonal changes, there is a natural decline in basal metabolic rate (BMR), the energy expended at rest. This decline can make it more challenging for menopausal women to maintain or lose weight, necessitating adjustments in dietary and lifestyle habits.

4. **Insulin Resistance:** Menopause is associated with an increased risk of insulin resistance, where cells become less responsive to the effects of insulin. Insulin resistance can lead to elevated blood sugar levels and an increased likelihood of developing metabolic conditions such as type 2 diabetes.

5. **Impact on Lipid Profile:** Hormonal changes during menopause can influence lipid metabolism. There is often an increase in low-density lipoprotein (LDL) cholesterol, commonly known as "bad" cholesterol, and a decrease in high-density

lipoprotein (HDL) cholesterol, or "good" cholesterol. These changes contribute to cardiovascular risk.

6. **Lifestyle Influences:** Lifestyle factors play a significant role in weight management and metabolic health during menopause. Sedentary behavior, poor dietary choices, and inadequate physical activity can exacerbate weight gain and metabolic disturbances. Conversely, adopting a healthy lifestyle can mitigate these effects.

- **Dietary Considerations:** Menopausal women should pay attention to their dietary choices to support metabolic health. A balanced diet rich in fruits, vegetables, lean proteins, and whole grains can provide essential nutrients while helping to manage weight and blood sugar levels.

- **Role of Physical Activity:** Regular physical activity is crucial for mitigating weight gain and supporting metabolic health during menopause. Both aerobic exercises and strength training contribute to calorie expenditure, muscle maintenance, and overall metabolic function.

- **Strength Training and Muscle Mass:** Strength training becomes particularly important during menopause as it helps preserve and build lean muscle mass. Since muscle tissue burns more calories at rest than fat tissue, maintaining muscle contributes to a higher metabolic rate.

- **Stress and Cortisol Levels:** Chronic stress during menopause can elevate cortisol levels, a hormone associated with increased abdominal fat deposition. Stress management techniques such as mindfulness, meditation, and adequate sleep can help mitigate the impact of stress on metabolism.

- **Adequate Sleep:** Quality sleep is integral to metabolic health. Sleep deprivation can disrupt hormonal balance, leading to increased appetite, cravings for high-calorie foods, and metabolic disturbances. Prioritizing adequate and restful sleep is crucial for weight management.

- **Hormone Replacement Therapy (HRT):** Hormone replacement therapy (HRT) may influence weight management in some menopausal women. Estrogen replacement can have varying effects on body composition, and the decision to undergo HRT should be made on an individual basis, considering potential risks and benefits.

- **Individual Variability:** It is essential to recognize the individual variability in the way menopause affects weight and metabolism. Factors such as genetics, pre-existing health conditions, and lifestyle choices contribute to the diversity of outcomes among menopausal women.

- **Preventive Strategies:** Proactive measures are key to managing weight and metabolic changes during and after menopause. A holistic approach that combines a healthy diet, regular physical activity, stress management, and, when appropriate, medical interventions can help women navigate this life stage with optimal metabolic well-being.

Breast Cancer Health

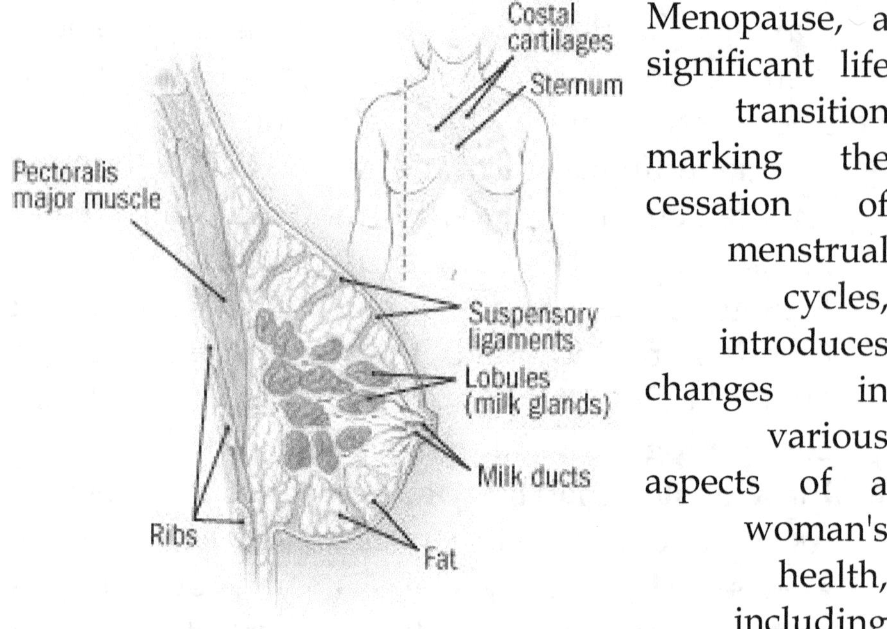

Menopause, a significant life transition marking the cessation of menstrual cycles, introduces changes in various aspects of a woman's health, including breast health. Understanding the nuances of breast health during menopause is essential for navigating potential risks and adopting proactive measures to ensure optimal well-being.

1. **Hormonal Influence on Breast Tissue:** Hormonal changes, particularly the decline in estrogen and progesterone during menopause, can influence breast tissue. Estrogen, in particular, plays a role in maintaining the density and structure of the breast. The hormonal fluctuations characteristic of menopause may impact breast tissue composition.
2. **Breast Cancer Risk:** Menopause is associated with an increased risk of breast cancer. The majority of breast cancers occur in women over the age of 50, and the risk continues to rise with age. Regular breast cancer screenings, such as mammograms, are crucial for early detection and intervention.
3. **Breast Density Changes:** Hormonal shifts can contribute to changes in breast density. As women progress through menopause, the density of breast tissue may decrease. However, dense breast tissue can make it more challenging to detect abnormalities on mammograms, highlighting the importance of regular screenings.
4. **Importance of Regular Breast Exams:** Self-examinations and clinical breast exams remain important components of breast health during menopause. Women are encouraged to be familiar with the normal look and feel of their breasts and promptly report any changes, such as lumps, to healthcare providers.

5. **Impact of Hormone Replacement Therapy (HRT):** The use of hormone replacement therapy (HRT) during menopause may influence breast health. While HRT can alleviate menopausal symptoms, it has been associated with a slight increase in breast cancer risk. Women considering HRT should discuss the potential risks and benefits with their healthcare providers.

6. **Lifestyle Factors and Breast Health:** Adopting a healthy lifestyle is crucial for promoting overall well-being, including breast health during menopause. Maintaining a balanced diet, engaging in regular physical activity, limiting alcohol consumption, and avoiding smoking contribute to holistic health and may reduce certain breast cancer risks.

7. **Bone Health and Breast Cancer Medications:** Medications prescribed for bone health, such as bisphosphonates, may have potential benefits in reducing the risk of certain types of breast cancer. However, individual considerations and discussions with healthcare providers are essential to determine the most appropriate course of action.

8. **Psychological Well-being and Breast Health:** The emotional and psychological aspects of menopause, including changes in body image and self-perception, can influence how women approach breast health. Open communication with

healthcare providers, regular check-ups, and emotional support contribute to holistic well-being.

- **Importance of Early Detection:** Early detection remains a cornerstone in managing breast health during menopause. Regular mammograms, breast exams, and an awareness of breast changes enable early intervention and improved outcomes in the event of a breast health concern.
- **Individualized Care and Healthcare Guidance:** Breast health is a highly individualized aspect of women's well-being, and healthcare guidance should be tailored to individual risk factors, health history, and preferences. Women should actively participate in discussions with their healthcare providers to make informed decisions.
- **Ongoing Monitoring and Education:** Ongoing monitoring of breast health and staying informed about the latest developments in breast cancer screening and prevention contribute to proactive care. Educational resources, support groups, and regular healthcare check-ups play integral roles in this ongoing process.

CHAPTER SIX

DIAGNOSTIC TOOLS AND TESTS

Hormone Levels Testing

Hormone levels testing is a valuable diagnostic tool used to assess the levels of various hormones in the body. This testing is particularly relevant in the context of menopause, where hormonal fluctuations play a central role in the physiological changes experienced by women.

Purpose and Significance:

Hormone levels testing is conducted to evaluate the concentration of specific hormones circulating in the bloodstream. This diagnostic tool is crucial for understanding the hormonal profile of an individual, identifying imbalances, and informing healthcare decisions, especially during life stages such as menopause.

Hormones Assessed:

Hormone panels for menopause often include assessments of key hormones, including:

- **Estrogen:** Various forms of estrogen, such as estradiol, estrone, and estriol, play pivotal roles in reproductive and overall health.
- **Progesterone:** Critical for the regulation of the menstrual cycle and maintenance of pregnancy.
- **Follicle-Stimulating Hormone (FSH):** Elevated FSH levels are indicative of diminished ovarian function and commonly used as a marker for menopause.
- **Luteinizing Hormone (LH):** Levels of LH often rise in conjunction with FSH during menopause.
- **Testosterone:** While often associated with males, women also produce testosterone, and its levels can influence aspects of women's health.

Indications for Testing:
Hormone levels testing is indicated in various situations, including:

- **Menopausal Symptoms:** Assessing hormone levels helps identify hormonal imbalances contributing to symptoms like hot flashes, mood swings, and sleep disturbances.
- **Menstrual Irregularities:** For women experiencing irregular menstrual cycles, hormone testing can provide insights into the underlying hormonal causes.

- **Fertility Assessment:** Hormone testing is employed to evaluate fertility, especially in cases of difficulty conceiving.
- **Monitoring Hormone Replacement Therapy (HRT):** For women undergoing HRT, regular hormone testing ensures appropriate hormone levels and treatment effectiveness.

Testing Methods:

Several methods are used for hormone levels testing:

- **Blood Tests:** The most common method involves drawing blood to measure hormone concentrations. This provides a snapshot of hormone levels at a specific moment.
- **Saliva Tests:** Saliva tests measure the "free" or unbound fraction of hormones. While convenient, their accuracy can be influenced by factors like recent food intake.
- **Urine Tests:** Urine tests may provide a more extended overview of hormone metabolites, offering insights into hormone processing and elimination.

Timing of Testing:

The timing of hormone testing is crucial, especially for assessing reproductive hormones like FSH and LH. In the context of menopause:

- **Day 3 FSH Test:** Often conducted on the third day of the menstrual cycle to assess ovarian function.
- **Mid-Cycle LH Surge:** To detect the surge in LH that precedes ovulation.
- **Random Estrogen and Progesterone Tests:** For women without regular menstrual cycles.

Interpreting Results:

Interpreting hormone test results requires expertise. Normal ranges vary, and healthcare providers consider individual factors, symptoms, and the specific hormones being assessed. Deviations from expected levels can guide further investigations and treatment decisions.

Limitations and Considerations:

Hormone levels testing, while informative, has limitations:

- **Variability:** Hormone levels can vary throughout the day and menstrual cycle.
- **Single Snapshot:** Blood tests offer a single snapshot and may not capture hormonal fluctuations adequately.
- **Individual Variability:** Normal hormone levels vary among individuals, and deviations do not necessarily imply pathology.

Integrated Approach to Menopause Management:

Hormone levels testing is one component of an integrated approach to menopause management. Healthcare providers use these results alongside clinical assessments, patient history, and symptomatology to tailor individualized treatment plans.

- Considerations for Hormone Replacement Therapy (HRT): For women considering or undergoing HRT, hormone levels testing is crucial for monitoring treatment efficacy and adjusting hormone dosages as needed.
- Patient Education and Empowerment: Patient education is paramount. Empowering individuals with knowledge about hormone testing, its purpose, and potential implications fosters informed decision-making and active participation in their healthcare.

Bone Density Scan

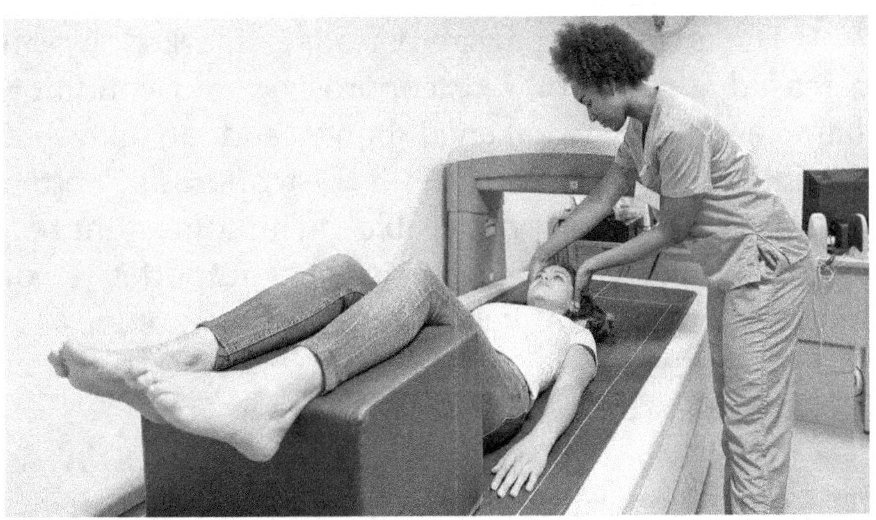

Bone density scans, often performed through Dual-Energy X-ray Absorptiometry (DEXA) scans, play a crucial role in assessing bone health, particularly in the context of menopause. Menopause is associated with hormonal changes that can impact bone density and increase the risk of osteoporosis. Here is a detailed exploration of the significance of bone density scans during menopause:

Hormonal Impact on Bone Health:

Menopause is characterized by a decline in estrogen levels. Estrogen plays a key role in maintaining bone density by regulating the activity of bone-forming cells (osteoblasts) and bone-resorbing cells (osteoclasts). The reduction in estrogen during menopause contributes to accelerated bone loss.

Osteoporosis Risk in Menopause:

The postmenopausal period is marked by an increased risk of osteoporosis, a condition characterized by weakened bones and an elevated susceptibility to fractures. Osteoporosis often progresses without noticeable symptoms until a fracture occurs, underscoring the importance of preventive measures such as bone density scans.

DEXA Scan:

Dual-Energy X-ray Absorptiometry (DEXA) is the gold standard for bone density assessment. It measures bone mineral density (BMD) at specific sites, commonly the hip and spine. The results are compared to the bone density of a young adult to determine T-scores, providing insights into bone health.

Timing of Bone Density Scans:

The timing of bone density scans during menopause is influenced by individual factors and risk profiles:

Baseline Scans: Women at the onset of menopause may undergo baseline bone density scans to assess initial bone health.

Follow-up Scans: Subsequent scans are often recommended based on individual risk factors, family history, and the results of initial scans.

Identification of Osteopenia and Osteoporosis:

DEXA scans classify bone health into three categories:

1. **Normal:** Bone density within the expected range for age.
2. **Osteopenia:** Lower than normal bone density, indicating bone weakening but not to the extent of osteoporosis.
3. **Osteoporosis:** Severe bone density loss, significantly increasing the risk of fractures.

Fracture Risk Assessment:

DEXA scans provide an estimate of fracture risk based on bone density measurements. This information guides healthcare providers in determining appropriate interventions, lifestyle modifications, and potential pharmacological treatments.

Integration with Clinical Assessment:

Bone density scans are an integral component of a comprehensive assessment that includes clinical evaluation, medical history, and risk factor analysis. This integrated approach informs personalized strategies for bone health management.

Lifestyle Measures and Bone Health:

Bone density scans guide the implementation of lifestyle measures to enhance bone health during menopause:

1. **Weight-Bearing Exercise:** Regular weight-bearing exercises, such as walking, jogging, and resistance training, promote bone density.
2. **Calcium and Vitamin D Intake:** Adequate calcium and vitamin D intake are essential for bone health. Supplements may be recommended based on individual dietary assessments.
3. **Smoking Cessation and Limiting Alcohol:** Smoking and excessive alcohol intake contribute to bone loss. Lifestyle modifications are encouraged for overall bone health.

Pharmacological Interventions:

In cases of significant bone loss or high fracture risk, healthcare providers may recommend pharmacological interventions. Medications, such as bisphosphonates, hormone therapy, or other bone-strengthening agents, are considered based on individual health considerations.

- **Follow-Up Monitoring:** Regular follow-up bone density scans are advised to monitor changes in bone health and assess the effectiveness of interventions. Adjustments to treatment plans can be made as needed.

- **Patient Education and Empowerment:** Patient education is crucial for fostering proactive bone health. Understanding the implications of bone density scans, lifestyle modifications, and the role of medical interventions empowers women to actively participate in their bone health management.
- **Holistic Approach to Bone Health:** Bone density scans are one aspect of a holistic approach to bone health during menopause. Combining medical assessments, lifestyle modifications, and ongoing monitoring ensures a comprehensive strategy for preserving bone density and reducing fracture risk.

Cardiovascular Risk Assessments

Menopause marks a significant life stage for women, characterized by hormonal changes that can influence cardiovascular health. As women transition through menopause, understanding and assessing cardiovascular risk becomes crucial for early intervention and prevention of heart-related complications.

Hormonal Changes and Cardiovascular Risk

Menopause involves a decline in estrogen levels, which can have implications for cardiovascular health. Estrogen, traditionally considered cardioprotective, plays a role in maintaining healthy blood vessels, regulating cholesterol levels, and influencing other factors that contribute to cardiovascular well-being.

Traditional Cardiovascular Risk Factors

Menopausal women are assessed for traditional cardiovascular risk factors, including:

1. **Hypertension:** Elevated blood pressure is a significant risk factor for cardiovascular diseases (CVD).
2. **Hyperlipidemia:** Abnormal levels of cholesterol, particularly high levels of low-density lipoprotein (LDL) cholesterol, contribute to atherosclerosis.
3. **Diabetes:** Women with diabetes have an increased risk of CVD.
4. **Smoking:** Tobacco use is a modifiable risk factor with profound effects on cardiovascular health.

Cardiovascular Risk Calculators

Various cardiovascular risk calculators, such as the Framingham Risk Score or the American College of Cardiology/American Heart Association (ACC/AHA) Risk Calculator, estimate the likelihood of experiencing a cardiovascular event over a specific time frame. These calculators consider age, blood pressure, cholesterol levels, smoking status, and other risk factors.

Unique Cardiovascular Considerations in Menopause

Menopause introduces unique considerations for cardiovascular risk assessments:

1. **Changes in Lipid Profile:** The decline in estrogen can lead to unfavorable changes in lipid profiles, including increased LDL cholesterol and decreased high-density lipoprotein (HDL) cholesterol.
2. **Weight Redistribution:** Hormonal changes may contribute to the redistribution of body fat, with an increased tendency for abdominal or visceral fat accumulation—a risk factor for cardiovascular disease.
3. **Blood Pressure Fluctuations:** Menopausal women may experience fluctuations in blood pressure, necessitating regular monitoring.

Imaging Studies for Cardiovascular Assessment:

Advanced imaging studies, such as coronary artery calcium scoring and carotid ultrasound, provide additional insights into cardiovascular health. These studies can detect the presence of arterial plaque and assess the risk of atherosclerosis.

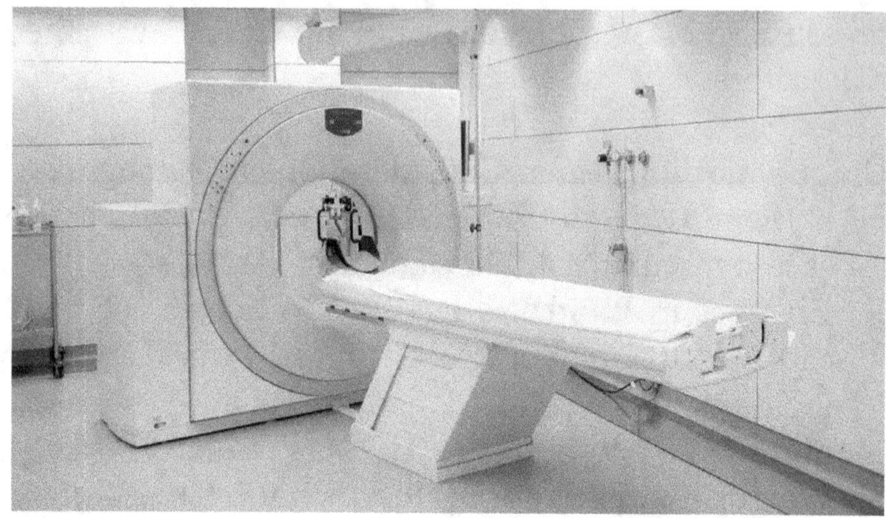

Coronary Artery Calcium Scoring

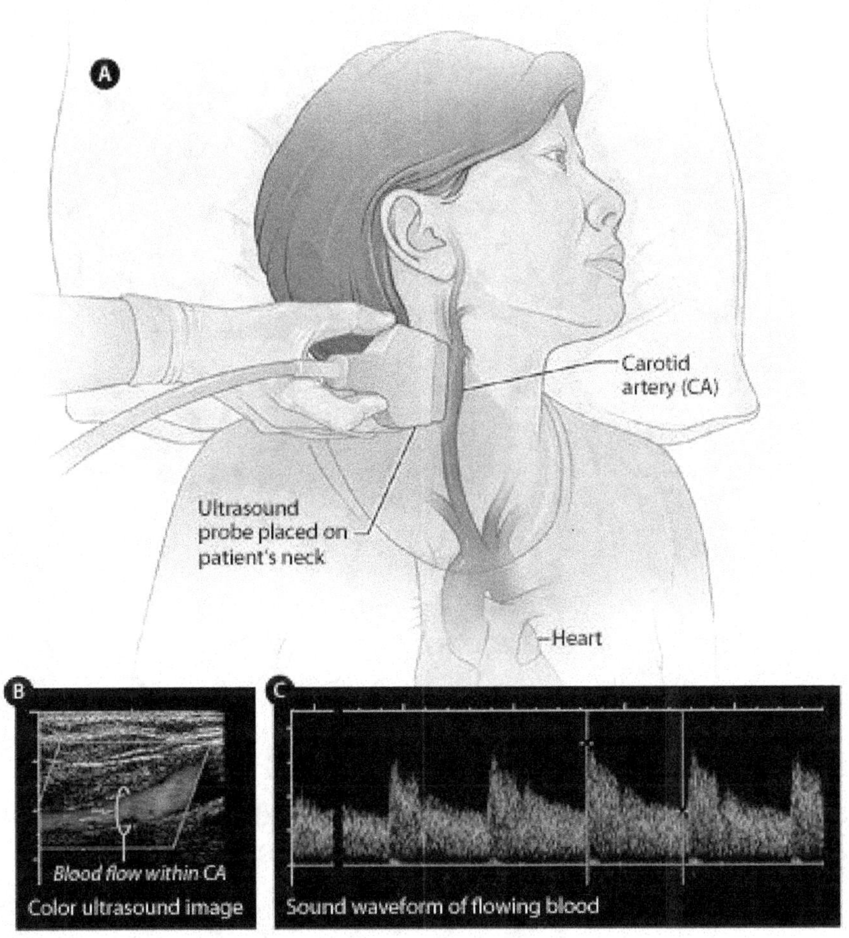

carotid ultrasound

Inflammatory Markers and Cardiovascular Risk

Inflammatory markers, such as C-reactive protein (CRP), are considered in cardiovascular risk assessments. Chronic inflammation is associated with atherosclerosis and contributes to cardiovascular risk.

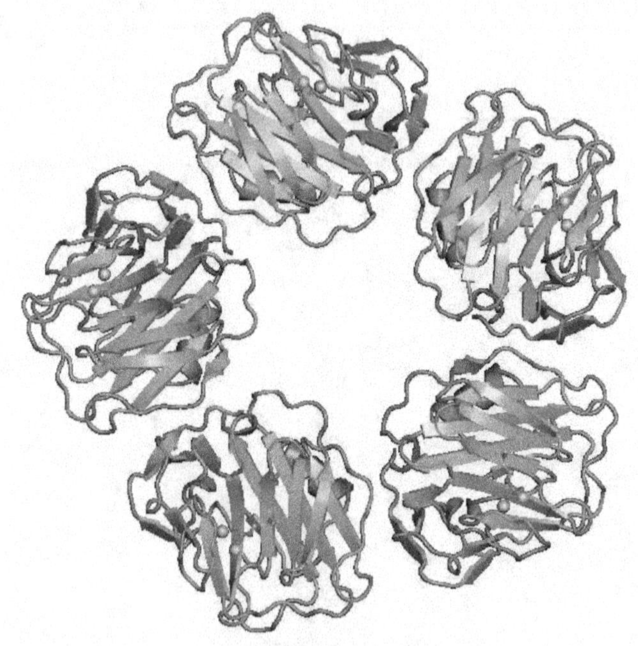

C-reactive protein

Lifestyle Factors and Cardiovascular Health

Lifestyle assessments are integral to cardiovascular risk evaluations:

1. **Dietary Habits:** A heart-healthy diet rich in fruits, vegetables, whole grains, and lean proteins is encouraged.

2. **Physical Activity:** Regular exercise contributes to cardiovascular fitness and weight management.

3. **Smoking and Alcohol Consumption:** Smoking cessation and moderation in alcohol intake are emphasized for overall cardiovascular health.

Hormone Replacement Therapy (HRT) and Cardiovascular Risk

The use of hormone replacement therapy (HRT) during menopause is a complex consideration. While it may alleviate menopausal symptoms, its impact on cardiovascular health is subject to ongoing research. Individualized assessments weigh potential risks and benefits.

- **Individualized Risk Assessments:** Cardiovascular risk assessments are individualized, considering each woman's unique health profile, family history, and lifestyle factors. This personalized approach allows for targeted interventions and optimal risk management.
- **Prevention and Intervention Strategies:** Based on risk assessments, prevention and intervention strategies are tailored to address specific cardiovascular risks. These may include lifestyle modifications, medication management, and ongoing monitoring.
- **Long-Term Monitoring:** Menopausal women undergo long-term monitoring of cardiovascular health. Regular assessments ensure the effectiveness of interventions and enable timely adjustments based on evolving risk profiles.

- **Patient Education and Empowerment:** Patient education is paramount for empowering women to actively participate in their cardiovascular health. Understanding risk factors, lifestyle modifications, and the importance of ongoing assessments fosters informed decision-making.

Breast Cancer Screenings

Breast cancer screenings are crucial components of women's healthcare, and their significance becomes even more pronounced during and after menopause. Menopause, characterized by hormonal changes, aging, and associated risk factors, necessitates a tailored approach to breast cancer prevention and early detection. Here's a detailed exploration of breast cancer screenings in relation to menopause:

Age and Breast Cancer Risk

The risk of breast cancer increases with age, and menopause marks a significant life stage where this risk becomes more prominent. Women over the age of 50 are at an elevated risk, emphasizing the importance of regular breast cancer screenings during and after menopause.

Mammography as the Gold Standard

Mammography is the gold standard for breast cancer screening. It involves X-ray imaging of the breast tissue to detect abnormalities, including tumors or microcalcifications. The American Cancer Society recommends annual mammograms for women starting at age 45, with the option to transition to biennial screenings at age 55.

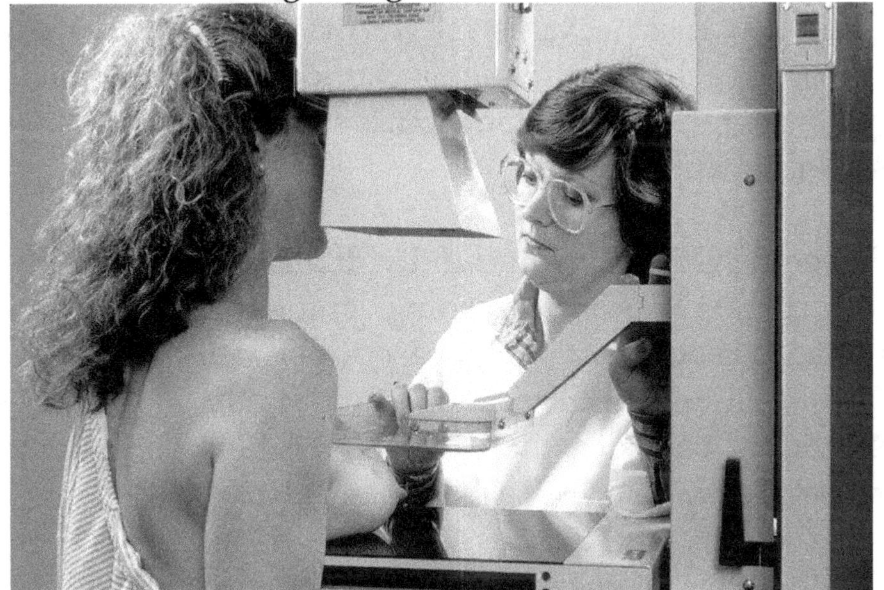

Mammography

Hormonal Changes and Breast Density

Menopausal hormonal changes impact breast density. Postmenopausal women often have less dense breast tissue, which can enhance the effectiveness of mammography in detecting abnormalities. However, hormone replacement therapy (HRT) can influence breast density, and its implications for screening are considered on an individual basis.

Breast Self-Exams and Clinical Breast Exams

While the emphasis on routine breast self-exams has evolved, women are still encouraged to be familiar with the normal look and feel of their breasts. Clinical breast exams performed by healthcare providers during regular check-ups complement mammography and contribute to a comprehensive screening approach.

Screening Guidelines and Individualized Approaches:

Breast cancer screening guidelines are often nuanced and may vary based on individual risk factors, family history, and health status. Healthcare providers consider these factors to tailor screening recommendations for each woman.

Digital Breast Tomosynthesis (DBT):

Digital breast tomosynthesis, or 3D mammography, is an advanced imaging technique that provides a three-dimensional view of the breast. It may offer improved cancer detection rates and reduce the need for additional imaging.

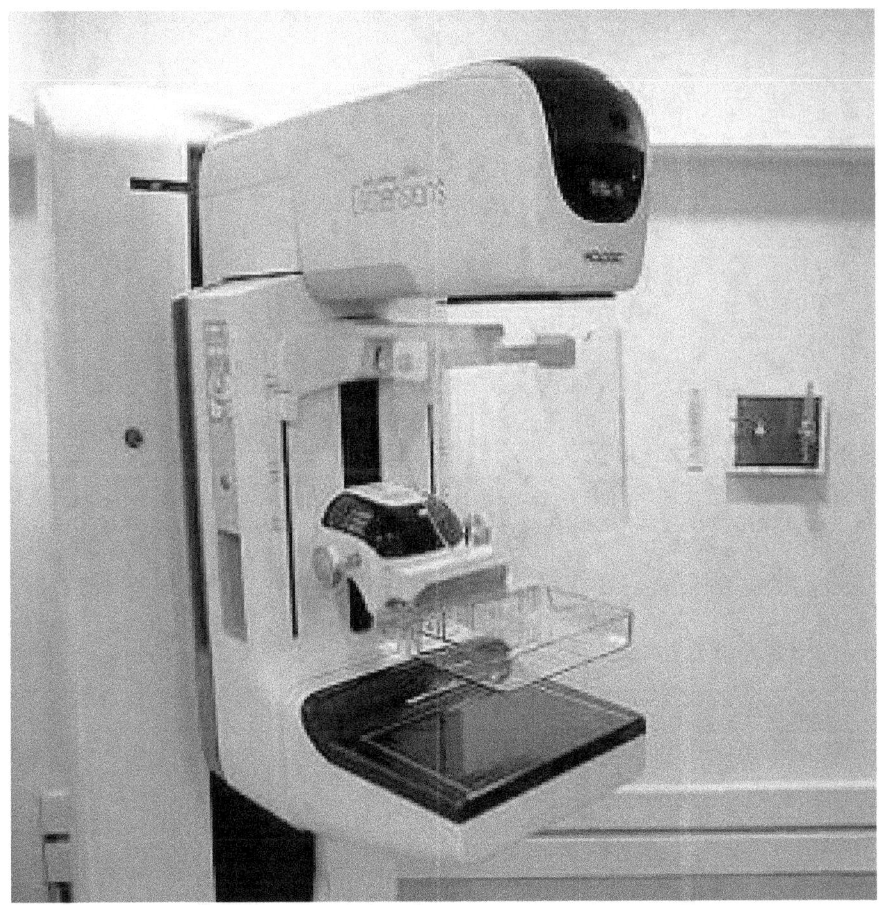

Digital Breast Tomosynthesis (DBT)

Breast Ultrasound and MRI

In certain cases, additional imaging modalities, such as breast ultrasound or magnetic resonance imaging (MRI), may be recommended. These techniques are particularly valuable for women with dense breast tissue or those at higher risk due to genetic factors.

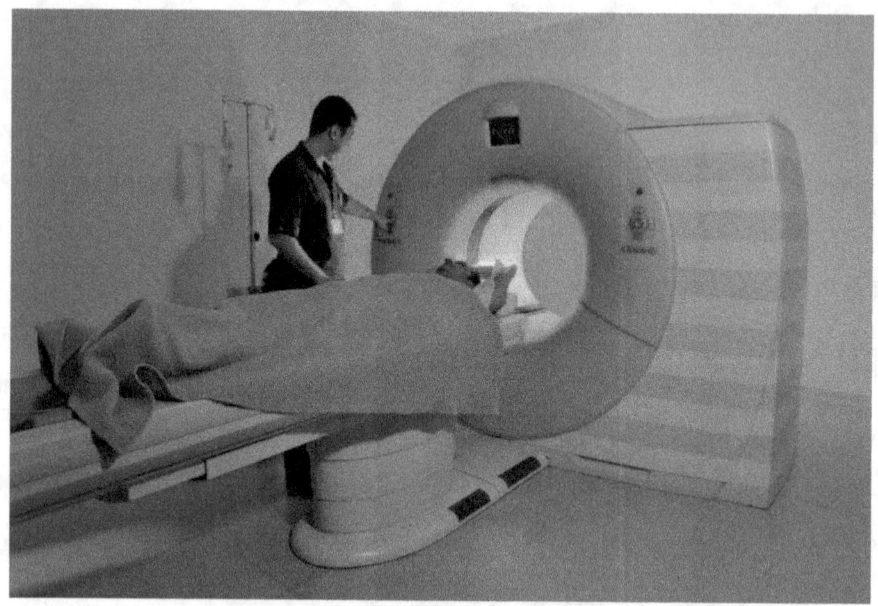

Magnetic Resonance Imaging (Mri)

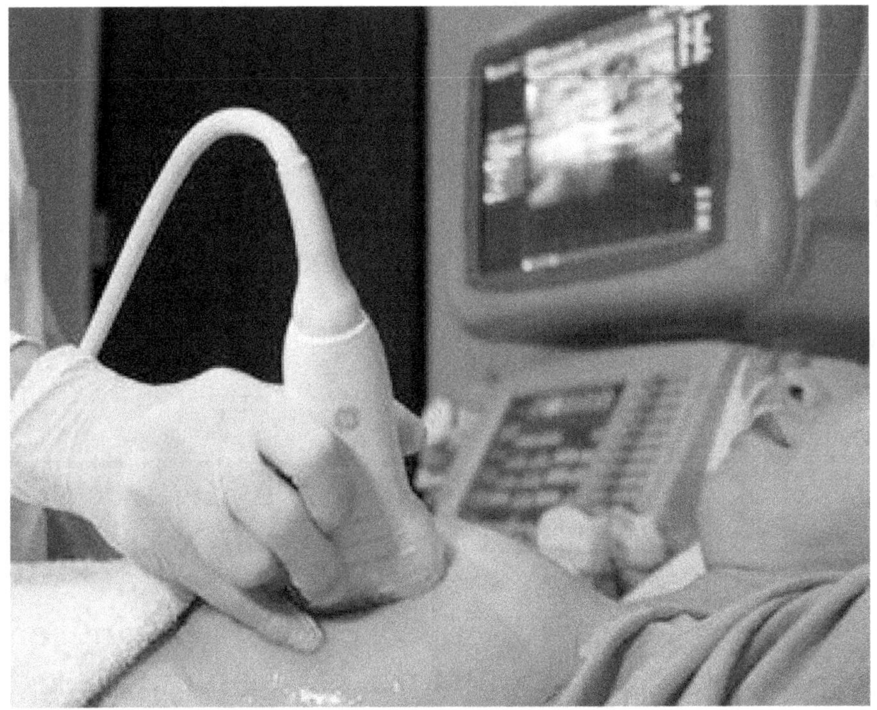

Breast Ultrasound

Genetic Testing and Counseling:

Women with a family history of breast cancer or specific genetic mutations may undergo genetic testing to assess their risk. Genetic counseling helps individuals make informed decisions about screenings, preventive measures, and potential interventions.

Personalized Risk Assessments:

Risk assessments, considering factors like family history, age, reproductive history, and hormonal influences, contribute to personalized breast cancer screening plans. Some women may benefit from earlier or more frequent screenings based on their individual risk profiles.

Breast Cancer Prevention Strategies:
1. Beyond screenings, women can adopt lifestyle strategies to reduce breast cancer risk during and after menopause:
2. **Healthy Diet:** A balanced diet rich in fruits, vegetables, and whole grains supports overall health.
3. **Regular Exercise:** Physical activity is associated with a lower risk of breast cancer and contributes to overall well-being.
4. **Limiting Alcohol:** Excessive alcohol consumption is linked to an increased risk of breast cancer, and moderation is advised.

- **Comprehensive Follow-Up and Communication:** Regular communication between women and their healthcare providers is crucial. Comprehensive follow-up, including discussions about screening results, potential interventions, and ongoing risk assessments, ensures a proactive approach to breast health.
- **Breast Cancer Awareness and Education:** Raising awareness about breast cancer, educating women about the importance of screenings, and promoting breast health literacy empower individuals to

actively participate in their healthcare and advocate for their well-being.

CHAPTER SEVEN

MANAGEMENT AND TREATMENT OPTIONS

Hormone Replacement Therapy (HRT)

Hormone Replacement Therapy (HRT) is a medical intervention designed to alleviate symptoms associated with hormonal changes, particularly those occurring during menopause. It involves the administration of hormones, often estrogen and progesterone, to restore hormonal balance and manage the physiological effects of hormonal decline.

Purpose of HRT
1. **Symptom Relief:** The primary purpose of HRT is to alleviate menopausal symptoms, including hot flashes, night sweats, vaginal dryness, and mood swings, by supplementing declining hormone levels.

Types of Hormones Used in HRT:
1. **Estrogen:** The most common hormone used in HRT. Estrogen can be administered in various forms, such as estradiol, estrone, and estriol.

2. **Progesterone:** If a woman has an intact uterus, progesterone is often prescribed alongside estrogen to reduce the risk of endometrial hyperplasia and cancer.
3. **Testosterone:** In some cases, testosterone may be included in HRT to address symptoms such as low libido and fatigue.

Forms of Administration
1. **Oral Tablets:** Estrogen and progesterone are commonly available in oral tablet form.
2. **Transdermal Patches or Gels:** These are applied to the skin, allowing for the gradual absorption of hormones.
3. **Vaginal Creams or Rings:** Used to address symptoms like vaginal dryness and discomfort.
4. **Injections or Implants:** Less common forms of administration.

Benefits of HRT
1. **Symptom Management:** Effectively alleviates menopausal symptoms, enhancing quality of life for many women.
2. **Bone Health:** Helps maintain bone density and reduces the risk of osteoporosis.
3. **Cardiovascular Health:** May have cardiovascular benefits, especially in the early postmenopausal period.

Risks and Considerations

1. **Breast Cancer Risk:** Long-term use of combined estrogen and progesterone therapy may be associated with a slightly increased risk of breast cancer. The relationship between HRT and breast cancer risk is complex and varies based on individual factors.
2. **Cardiovascular Risks:** The impact of HRT on cardiovascular health is subject to ongoing research and may vary based on factors such as age, health status, and the specific hormones used.
3. **Thromboembolism:** HRT may increase the risk of blood clots, particularly in the legs (deep vein thrombosis) or lungs (pulmonary embolism).
4. **Stroke:** Some studies suggest a slight increase in the risk of stroke associated with HRT, especially in older women.
5. **Endometrial Cancer:** The use of estrogen alone in women with an intact uterus may increase the risk of endometrial cancer. Adding progesterone helps mitigate this risk.

Individualized Treatment Plans:

HRT decisions should be individualized based on a woman's health history, symptoms, and risk factors. Healthcare providers consider factors such as age, overall health, family history, and personal preferences when recommending HRT.

Timing and Duration
The timing of initiating HRT is a crucial consideration. Starting closer to the onset of menopause may provide more significant symptom relief. The duration of HRT use is also individualized, with ongoing assessments to evaluate the ongoing benefits and risks.

Alternatives to HRT
1. **Lifestyle Modifications:** Healthy diet, regular exercise, and stress management can help alleviate menopausal symptoms.
2. **Non-Hormonal Medications:** Certain medications, such as selective serotonin reuptake inhibitors (SSRIs) and selective norepinephrine reuptake inhibitors (SNRIs), can be effective for managing hot flashes.
3. **Herbal Supplements:** Some women explore herbal remedies like black cohosh or soy products, although their efficacy varies.

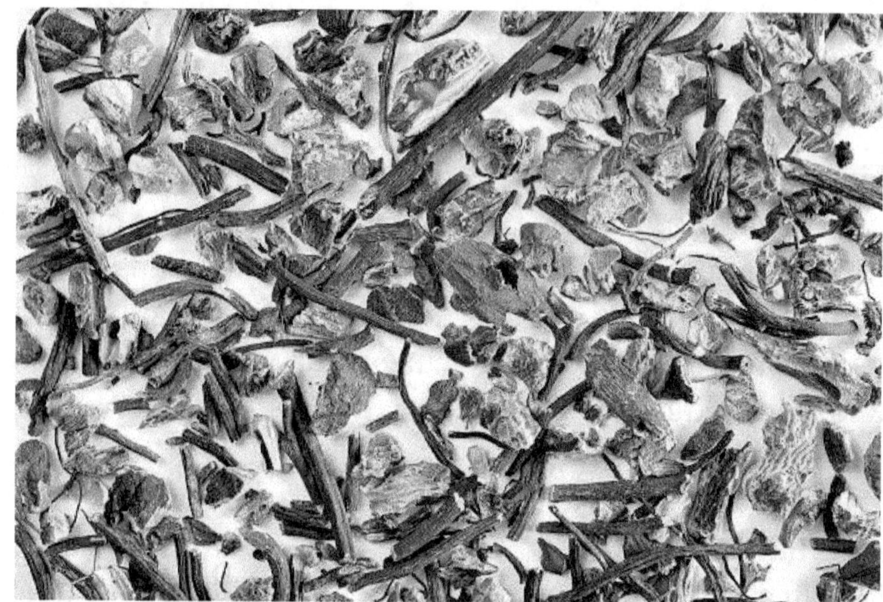

Black Cohosh

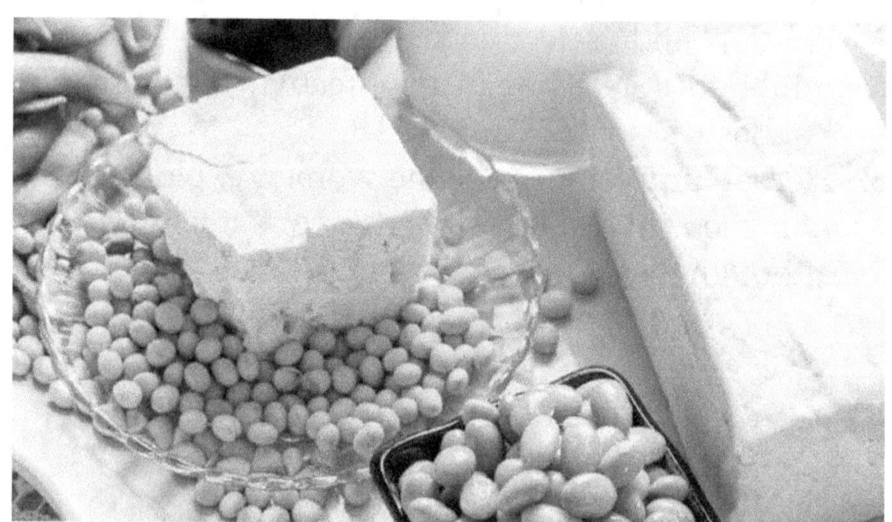

Soy Products

- **Regular Monitoring and Follow-Up:** Women on HRT require regular monitoring. Follow-up appointments with healthcare providers ensure that the treatment plan is effective, and any emerging concerns are addressed promptly.
- **Shared Decision-Making:** Decision-making regarding HRT involves collaboration between the woman and her healthcare provider. Open communication, informed discussions, and ongoing assessments contribute to a shared decision-making process.
- **Impact on Quality of Life:** For many women, HRT can significantly improve the quality of life during the menopausal transition. It addresses bothersome symptoms and supports overall well-being.
- **Emerging Research and Evolving Guidelines:** HRT research is dynamic, and guidelines may evolve based on new evidence. Women and healthcare providers should stay informed about the latest research findings and guidelines to make informed decisions.

Non-Hormonal Pharmacological Interventions

Menopause, a natural phase marking the end of reproductive years, is associated with hormonal changes that can lead to a range of symptoms. While hormone replacement therapy (HRT) is one option for managing these symptoms, some women may seek non-hormonal pharmacological interventions. These interventions aim to alleviate menopausal symptoms without the use of hormones.

Antidepressants and Mood Stabilizers:

1. **Selective Serotonin Reuptake Inhibitors (SSRIs) and Serotonin-Norepinephrine Reuptake Inhibitors (SNRIs):** Medications like fluoxetine, venlafaxine, or duloxetine are commonly used to address mood swings, irritability, and anxiety during menopause.

Gabapentin and Pregabalin

These anticonvulsant medications may be prescribed to manage hot flashes. They are thought to modulate the central nervous system and reduce the frequency and intensity of hot flashes.

Clonidine

Originally used for hypertension, clonidine has been found to be effective in reducing hot flashes. Its mechanism of action involves influencing the central nervous system's regulation of body temperature.

Antiepileptic Medications

Some antiepileptic drugs, such as topiramate, have shown efficacy in reducing the frequency and severity of hot flashes. Their exact mechanism in addressing menopausal symptoms is still under investigation.

Ospemifene

Opemifene is a selective estrogen receptor modulator (SERM) that acts selectively on estrogen receptors. It is used to address vulvovaginal atrophy, a common concern during menopause, without stimulating the endometrium.

Gabapentin Enacarbil

Similar to gabapentin, this extended-release form is used to manage moderate to severe hot flashes associated with menopause.

Duavee (Conjugated Estrogen/Bazedoxifene)

Duavee combines conjugated estrogen with bazedoxifene, a selective estrogen receptor modulator. It is used to alleviate vasomotor symptoms (hot flashes) and prevent postmenopausal osteoporosis without stimulating the endometrium.

Nonsteroidal Anti-Inflammatory Drugs (NSAIDs)

NSAIDs may be recommended for managing pain and discomfort associated with conditions like osteoarthritis, which can be exacerbated during the menopausal years.

Bisphosphonates

While primarily used for managing osteoporosis, bisphosphonates like alendronate may be prescribed during menopause to address bone density concerns.

Cognitive Behavioral Therapy (CBT): While not pharmacological, CBT is a psychological intervention that has demonstrated effectiveness in managing mood symptoms and improving sleep quality during menopause.

Lifestyle Modifications:

Lifestyle changes are integral to managing menopausal symptoms:

1. **Regular Exercise:** Physical activity contributes to overall well-being, helps manage weight, and can alleviate mood swings and insomnia.

2. **Healthy Diet:** A balanced diet rich in nutrients supports general health and may help manage symptoms.
3. **Stress Reduction Techniques:** Practices such as mindfulness, meditation, and yoga can help alleviate stress and improve mental well-being.
4. **Adequate Sleep:** Establishing healthy sleep habits is crucial for managing insomnia and promoting overall health.

Phytoestrogens

While not strictly pharmacological, some women turn to plant-derived compounds like soy isoflavones or black cohosh, which have estrogen-like effects and may help manage certain menopausal symptoms.

Vaginal Moisturizers and Lubricants

For addressing vaginal dryness and discomfort, non-hormonal moisturizers and lubricants can provide relief. They are applied topically and help maintain vaginal health.

Complementary and Alternative Medicine (CAM)

Some women explore CAM options, including herbal supplements like evening primrose oil, dong quai, or red clover. However, the efficacy and safety of these supplements are not universally established, and caution is advised.

Individualized Approach

The choice of non-hormonal pharmacological interventions should be individualized, taking into account the woman's overall health, specific symptoms, and preferences. Regular communication with healthcare providers is crucial to assess efficacy and adjust treatment plans as needed

Lifestyle Modifications

Menopause, a natural and transformative phase in a woman's life, introduces hormonal changes that can impact physical, emotional, and mental well-being. While medical interventions exist, integrating lifestyle modifications is a proactive and comprehensive strategy to manage menopausal symptoms and enhance overall health. Here's an in-depth exploration of lifestyle modifications as integral components of menopause management:

1. **Regular Exercise:** Engaging in regular physical activity is paramount during menopause. Exercise helps maintain a healthy weight, improves mood, and supports bone health. Weight-bearing exercises, such as walking, jogging, or strength

training, are particularly beneficial for preserving bone density, which tends to decline during menopause. Additionally, cardiovascular exercises enhance heart health and contribute to overall fitness.

2. **Balanced Nutrition:** A well-balanced diet is essential for managing menopausal symptoms. Adequate intake of calcium and vitamin D supports bone health, reducing the risk of osteoporosis. Including a variety of fruits, vegetables, whole grains, and lean proteins helps maintain a healthy weight and provides essential nutrients. Omega-3 fatty acids, found in fish, flaxseeds, and walnuts, may help alleviate mood swings and support heart health.

3. **Hydration:** Staying well-hydrated is crucial, especially considering the potential increase in hot flashes and night sweats during menopause. Adequate water intake supports overall health and can help manage symptoms like dry skin and vaginal dryness.

4. **Stress Management:** Chronic stress can exacerbate menopausal symptoms and impact overall well-being. Incorporating stress management techniques, such as mindfulness, meditation, or

deep breathing exercises, can help alleviate stress and promote emotional balance. Finding activities that bring joy and relaxation, such as hobbies or spending time in nature, contributes to a positive mindset.

5. **Adequate Sleep:** Menopausal women often experience disruptions in sleep patterns, including insomnia or frequent awakenings. Establishing a consistent sleep routine, creating a comfortable sleep environment, and avoiding stimulants like caffeine before bedtime can contribute to better sleep quality. If sleep disturbances persist, consulting a healthcare professional is advisable.

6. **Limiting Alcohol and Caffeine:** Both alcohol and caffeine can contribute to exacerbating symptoms such as hot flashes and sleep disturbances. Limiting the intake of these substances, especially in the evening, may help manage symptoms and improve overall health.

7. **Quit Smoking:** Smoking is associated with an increased risk of cardiovascular issues and osteoporosis, conditions that menopausal women may be more susceptible to. Quitting smoking not only benefits overall health but can also reduce the severity of certain menopausal symptoms.

8. **Social Connections:** Maintaining strong social connections is crucial during menopause. The emotional support from friends and family can help alleviate feelings of isolation and contribute to a positive outlook. Joining support groups or participating in social activities can provide a sense of community and understanding.

9. **Mind-Body Practices:** Integrating mind-body practices such as yoga or tai chi can be beneficial for both physical and mental well-being. These practices combine gentle physical activity with mindfulness, promoting relaxation and stress reduction.

10. **Regular Health Check-ups:** Regular health check-ups with healthcare professionals, including gynecologists and primary care physicians, are essential during menopause. Monitoring cholesterol levels, bone density, and addressing any emerging health concerns in a timely manner is crucial for overall health.

11. **Maintaining a Positive Body Image:** Menopause often brings about changes in body composition and appearance. Embracing these changes and maintaining a positive body image is vital for

psychological well-being. Engaging in activities that promote self-love and self-care can contribute to a positive sense of self.

Integrative And Complementary Therapies

Integrative and complementary therapies offer a holistic approach to menopause management, focusing on enhancing well-being and alleviating symptoms through a combination of conventional and alternative methods. Here's a detailed exploration of integrative and complementary therapies in the context of menopause:

1. **Understanding Integrative and Complementary Therapies:**
- **Definition:** Integrative and complementary therapies refer to approaches that combine conventional medical treatments with alternative or holistic practices to address physical, emotional, and spiritual aspects of health.
- **Holistic Approach:** These therapies recognize the interconnectedness of mind, body, and spirit, aiming to promote overall well-being rather than simply treating specific symptoms.

2. Herbal Remedies and Supplements:

- **Black Cohosh:**

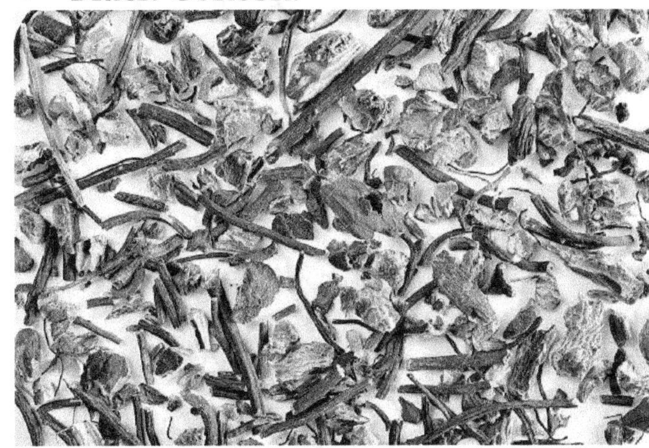

Widely used for managing menopausal symptoms, black cohosh may help alleviate hot flashes and night sweats.

- **Soy Isoflavones:**

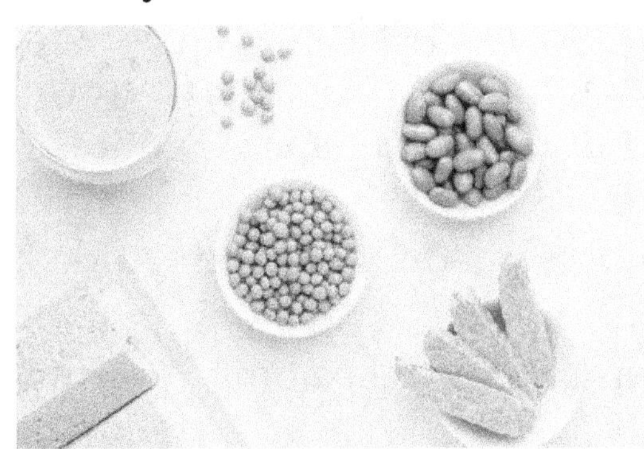

Rich in phytoestrogens, soy isoflavones may provide a natural alternative to hormone therapy in managing hormonal fluctuations.

- **Red Clover:**

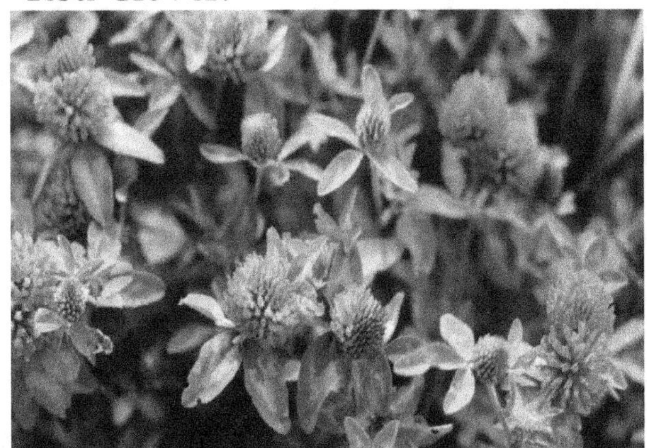

Contains compounds with estrogen-like effects,

potentially easing menopausal symptoms.

3. **Acupuncture:**
*   **Procedure:** Acupuncture involves inserting thin needles into specific points on the body to stimulate energy flow. It is used to address various menopausal symptoms, including hot flashes and sleep disturbances.
*   **Benefits:** Some women report reduced frequency and intensity of hot flashes, improved sleep, and enhanced overall well-being.

4. **Yoga and Meditation:**
*   **Yoga:** Combines physical postures, breathing exercises, and meditation. It may help reduce stress, improve flexibility, and enhance emotional well-being.
*   **Meditation:** Mindfulness meditation and guided imagery can be effective in managing stress, anxiety, and promoting relaxation during menopause.

5. **Massage Therapy:**
*   **Techniques:** Various massage techniques, including Swedish massage and aromatherapy, can promote relaxation and alleviate muscle tension associated with menopausal symptoms.

- **Benefits:** Improved sleep, reduced anxiety, and enhanced mood are reported benefits of regular massage therapy.

6. **Mind-Body Techniques:**
- **Biofeedback:** Involves learning to control physiological functions to reduce stress and manage symptoms like hot flashes.
- **Hypnotherapy:** Uses guided relaxation and focused attention to help manage symptoms such as insomnia and anxiety.

7. **Chiropractic Care:**
- **Approach:** Chiropractic care focuses on the musculoskeletal system, aiming to enhance overall health by addressing spinal misalignments.
- **Benefits:** Some women find relief from musculoskeletal discomfort and improved overall well-being with chiropractic adjustments.

8. **Traditional Chinese Medicine (TCM):**
- **Herbal Medicine:** TCM often incorporates herbal remedies to address imbalances and promote overall health during menopause.
- **Acupuncture:** Integral to TCM, acupuncture is used to balance energy flow and address specific symptoms.

9. **Dietary and Nutritional Approaches:**
- **Supplements:** Beyond herbal remedies, supplements like calcium and vitamin D are often recommended for bone health during and after menopause.
- **Nutrition Counseling:** Tailoring the diet to individual needs, including managing weight and incorporating nutrient-dense foods, contributes to overall health.

10. **Aromatherapy:**
- **Essential Oils:** Certain essential oils, such as lavender and peppermint, are used in aromatherapy to promote relaxation and alleviate symptoms like insomnia and stress.
- **Application:** Oils can be diffused, applied topically, or added to bathwater.

11. **Homeopathy:**
- **Principles:** Homeopathy involves using highly diluted substances to stimulate the body's self-healing abilities.
- **Individualized Treatment:** Homeopathic remedies are selected based on the unique symptoms and constitution of each individual.

12. **Balancing Hormones with Bioidentical Hormone Therapy (BHT):**

- **Definition:** BHT involves the use of hormones that are chemically identical to those produced by the body.
- **Considerations:** BHT is a controversial therapy, and its safety and efficacy should be thoroughly discussed with healthcare providers.

13. Consulting Healthcare Providers:

- **Integration with Conventional Care:** It is crucial to inform healthcare providers about any integrative or complementary therapies being pursued to ensure they complement rather than interfere with conventional treatments.
- **Individualized Approaches:** Healthcare providers can help tailor an integrative approach to menopause management based on individual health profiles and preferences.

14. Research and Evidence:

- **Varied Evidence:** The evidence supporting the effectiveness of integrative and complementary therapies varies. While some women find significant relief, individual responses can differ.
- **Informed Decision-Making:** Women are encouraged to research therapies, consult with healthcare providers, and make informed decisions based on their unique needs and preferences.

CHAPTER EIGHT

POST-MENOPAUSE: EMBRACING A NEW PHASE

Definition and Characteristics

Definition of Post-Menopause: Post-menopause is a distinct phase in a woman's life that follows the completion of the menopausal transition. It is officially recognized when a woman has not experienced menstruation for a consecutive 12-month period, signifying the cessation of reproductive capabilities. This phase typically begins around the age of 51, but the timing can vary widely among individuals. Post-menopause marks the conclusion of the hormonal fluctuations and reproductive changes associated with menopause, bringing about a more stabilized hormonal profile.

Characteristics of Post-Menopause:
1. **Absence of Menstruation:** Post-menopause is officially recognized after a continuous absence of menstruation for 12 consecutive months. This marks the conclusion of the reproductive phase, signifying a biological shift.

2. **Stable Hormone Levels:** Hormonally, post-menopausal women experience consistently low levels of estrogen and progesterone. Hormonal fluctuations, prevalent during perimenopause, subside, resulting in a more stable hormonal environment.

3. **Physical Changes:** Post-menopausal women may undergo physical changes, including alterations in skin elasticity, hair texture, and nail strength. A notable concern is the potential decline in bone density, leading to an increased risk of osteoporosis. Adequate calcium and vitamin D intake, coupled with weight-bearing exercises, become crucial for maintaining bone health.

4. **Cardiovascular Health:** Changes in cardiovascular health are observed during post-menopause, with a heightened risk of cardiovascular diseases due to reduced estrogen levels. Embracing a heart-healthy lifestyle, encompassing regular exercise and a balanced diet, becomes imperative to manage this risk effectively.

5. **Genitourinary Changes:** Post-menopausal symptoms often include vaginal dryness and thinning of vaginal walls attributed to decreased estrogen levels. These changes may result in discomfort during sexual intercourse and an elevated risk of urinary tract infections, requiring

interventions such as vaginal moisturizers or lubricants.

6. **Metabolic Changes:** Metabolically, post-menopausal women may experience shifts, including a propensity for weight gain, particularly around the abdominal area. Maintaining a healthy weight through a balanced diet and regular exercise becomes pivotal for managing metabolic changes.

7. **Mood and Mental Health:** While hormonal fluctuations during menopause influence mood, post-menopausal women often report improved emotional well-being. The stabilization of hormonal levels contributes to a sense of emotional balance. Nevertheless, external factors such as stress and lifestyle choices continue to impact mental health.

8. **Gynecological Health:** Prioritizing gynecological health remains crucial during post-menopause. Women are advised to sustain regular screenings, encompassing Pap smears and mammograms, to monitor for signs of gynecological cancers. Regular pelvic exams aid in assessing gynecological health, necessitating open communication with healthcare providers regarding any concerns.

9. **Hormone Replacement Therapy (HRT):** Some women may opt for hormone replacement therapy (HRT) during post-menopause to manage

symptoms like hot flashes, vaginal dryness, and mood swings. Decisions regarding HRT should be individualized, accounting for overall health, personal preferences, and potential risks and benefits.

10. **Healthy Lifestyle Choices:** Healthy lifestyle choices assume increasing importance during post-menopause. Regular exercise, a balanced diet, and effective stress management contribute significantly to overall well-being. Attention to cardiovascular health, bone health, and mental well-being through lifestyle adjustments and periodic health check-ups becomes paramount.

11. **Sexual Health:** Sexual health may undergo changes, with post-menopausal women experiencing shifts in sexual desire and response. Open communication with healthcare providers and, when necessary, sex therapists can address concerns related to sexual health and intimacy.

12. **Empowerment and Self-Care:** Post-menopause presents an opportunity for women to prioritize self-care and empowerment. Embracing the positive aspects of this life stage, such as freedom from menstrual cycles and potential relief from certain menopausal symptoms, contributes to a positive outlook and enhanced well-being.

Embracing the Post-Menopausal Phase:

1. **Understanding the Transition:** Acknowledging the post-menopausal phase involves recognizing it as a natural and inevitable part of the aging process. Understanding that hormonal changes are occurring and appreciating the significance of this transition lays the foundation for embracing the subsequent stage.

2. **Shifting Perspectives:** Embracing post-menopause requires a shift in perspectives regarding aging and self-image. Women can choose to view this phase as a time of wisdom, experience, and newfound freedom rather than solely as a marker of physical changes.

3. **Self-Care and Wellness:** Prioritizing self-care becomes essential during post-menopause. This includes adopting a holistic approach to wellness, encompassing regular exercise, a balanced diet, sufficient sleep, and stress management. Nurturing physical and mental well-being contributes to an overall positive experience of this life stage.

4. **Healthy Lifestyle Choices:** Embracing post-menopause involves making conscious and healthy lifestyle choices. Regular physical activity, such as aerobic exercises and strength training, supports cardiovascular health and helps maintain bone density. A nutritious diet rich in calcium and vitamin D contributes to overall health and addresses specific post-menopausal concerns.

5. **Mind-Body Practices:** Integrating mind-body practices, such as yoga or meditation, can be beneficial for managing stress and promoting emotional well-being. These practices offer a holistic approach that addresses both the physical and mental aspects of post-menopause.

6. **Sexual Well-Being:** Open communication about sexual health and intimacy is crucial during this phase. Embracing changes in sexual desire and response, along with discussing concerns with healthcare providers, can lead to a more fulfilling and satisfying post-menopausal experience.

7. **Continued Gynecological Health:** Embracing post-menopause involves a commitment to continued gynecological health. Regular screenings for gynecological cancers, such as Pap smears and mammograms, remain important. Maintaining open communication with healthcare providers ensures proactive management of any emerging health concerns.

8. **Positive Body Image:** Fostering a positive body image is integral to embracing post-menopause. Celebrating the body's resilience and appreciating it for its capabilities can contribute to improved self-esteem and overall satisfaction with one's physical self.

9. **Community and Support:** Building a supportive community and seeking emotional support from

friends, family, or support groups can be beneficial. Sharing experiences and learning from others navigating the post-menopausal phase fosters a sense of camaraderie and understanding.

10. **Mindset and Empowerment:** Cultivating a positive mindset and embracing empowerment are central to navigating post-menopause successfully. Women can view this phase as an opportunity to redefine priorities, pursue personal goals, and embrace newfound freedoms.

11. **Education and Awareness:** Staying informed about the changes associated with post-menopause and seeking reliable information is empowering. Understanding the physical and emotional aspects of this stage enables women to make informed decisions about their health and well-being.

12. **Celebrating Achievements:** Embracing post-menopause involves celebrating personal and professional achievements. Recognizing one's resilience, accomplishments, and the wisdom gained over the years contributes to a positive and fulfilling post-menopausal experience.

Persistence of Symptoms

Post-menopause, typically defined as the phase following 12 consecutive months without menstruation, is expected to bring relief from the often challenging symptoms of menopause. However, for some women, certain symptoms persist, requiring attention and management. Understanding the persistence of these symptoms is crucial for women's health and well-being during this life stage.

Hormonal Changes and Symptomatology:
1. **Estrogen Decline:** The hormonal fluctuations that characterize menopause, particularly the decline in estrogen levels, can contribute to persistent symptoms.
2. **Individual Variations:** Hormonal changes affect women differently, leading to a spectrum of experiences. Some women may continue to experience symptoms while others find relief.

Common Persistent Symptoms:
a. Hot Flashes and Night Sweats:
- **Cause:** Fluctuating hormone levels, particularly estrogen, can trigger hot flashes and night sweats.
- **Management:** Lifestyle modifications, hormone therapy, or non-hormonal medications may be considered for symptom relief.
b. Vaginal Dryness and Discomfort:
- **Cause:** Declining estrogen levels result in changes to the vaginal tissues, leading to dryness and discomfort.

- **Management:** Vaginal moisturizers, lubricants, and hormonal treatments may help alleviate symptoms and improve sexual health.

c. **Sleep Disturbances:**

- **Cause:** Hormonal changes, coupled with other factors like stress or lifestyle, can contribute to ongoing sleep issues.
- **Management:** Sleep hygiene practices, relaxation techniques, and, if necessary, medical interventions may be explored.

d. **Mood Swings and Emotional Well-being:**

- **Cause:** Hormonal fluctuations and life transitions can impact mood and emotional well-being.
- **Management:** Counseling, support groups, mindfulness practices, and sometimes medication can contribute to emotional balance.

e. **Joint Pain and Muscular Discomfort:**

- **Cause:** Changes in collagen production and joint lubrication due to hormonal changes may result in joint pain.
- **Management:** Exercise, joint-friendly activities, and, if needed, pain management strategies can help address discomfort.

Individual Variability:

- **Genetic Factors:** Individual genetic makeup can influence how women experience and manage post-menopausal symptoms.

- **Health History:** Pre-existing health conditions and lifestyle factors contribute to the variability of symptoms.

Impact on Quality of Life:
- **Physical Discomfort:** Persistent symptoms can affect daily activities, sleep quality, and overall physical comfort.
- **Emotional Toll:** Chronic symptoms may take an emotional toll, impacting mental health and quality of life.

Management and Treatment Options:
a.   Hormone Therapy:
- **Benefits:** For some women, hormone therapy can effectively alleviate persistent symptoms by supplementing declining estrogen levels.
- **Considerations:** Risks and benefits should be thoroughly discussed with healthcare providers, considering individual health profiles.

b.   Non-Hormonal Medications:
- **Antidepressants:** Some medications, such as selective serotonin reuptake inhibitors (SSRIs), may help manage symptoms like hot flashes.
- **Gabapentin:** This medication may be considered for its efficacy in reducing hot flashes and improving sleep.

c.   Lifestyle Modifications:

- **Diet and Nutrition:** Adopting a well-balanced diet rich in nutrients can contribute to overall health and symptom management.
- **Exercise:** Regular physical activity has been shown to alleviate symptoms and improve well-being.
- **Stress Management:** Techniques like mindfulness, meditation, and relaxation exercises can help manage stress-related symptoms.

d.　　Complementary Therapies:

- **Acupuncture:** Some women find relief from symptoms through acupuncture sessions.
- **Herbal Supplements:** Certain herbs, like black cohosh and soy, are believed to have potential benefits for symptom management.

Healthcare Provider Collaboration:
- **Individualized Approach:** Collaborating with healthcare providers is essential for developing personalized management plans.
- **Regular Check-ups:** Ongoing monitoring of symptoms, health status, and any potential side effects from treatments ensures effective and safe management.

Psychological Support:
- **Counseling and Support Groups:** Emotional well-being is integral to symptom management.

Counseling or participation in support groups can provide valuable coping strategies.

Research and Advancements:
- **Ongoing Studies:** The medical community continues to research and explore new approaches to managing persistent post-menopausal symptoms.
- **Clinical Trials:** Participation in clinical trials may provide women with access to cutting-edge treatments and therapies.

Health Risks In Post-Menopause

Post-menopause is a transformative phase in a woman's life characterized by the cessation of menstrual cycles and significant hormonal changes. While it marks the end of the reproductive years, it also brings about health considerations that merit careful attention. Understanding the health risks associated with post-menopause is crucial for women and their healthcare providers to implement effective preventive strategies and ensure optimal well-being.

Cardiovascular Health
1. **Risk of Heart Disease:**
a. **Estrogen Decline:** Post-menopausal women face an increased risk of heart disease due to the decline in

estrogen levels, which previously provided protective cardiovascular effects.

b. **Atherosclerosis:** The risk of atherosclerosis, characterized by the buildup of plaque in arteries, rises post-menopause, contributing to heart-related complications.

2. Hypertension:

a. **Incidence Increase:** Post-menopausal women may experience an elevated risk of hypertension. Regular monitoring of blood pressure and lifestyle modifications are crucial for prevention.

3. Lipid Profile Changes:

a. **Altered Lipid Levels:** Changes in lipid profiles, including an increase in LDL cholesterol and a decrease in HDL cholesterol, contribute to cardiovascular risks. Dietary adjustments and regular lipid screenings are essential.

Bone Health

1. Osteoporosis:

a. **Estrogen's Role:** With declining estrogen levels, post-menopausal women are at an increased risk of osteoporosis. This condition leads to weakened bones, making fractures more likely.

b. **Preventive Measures:** Calcium and vitamin D supplementation, weight-bearing exercises, and bone density scans help in preventing and managing osteoporosis.

Metabolic Changes

1. **Insulin Resistance:**

a. **Metabolic Shifts:** Post-menopause can lead to metabolic changes, including insulin resistance. This contributes to an increased risk of type 2 diabetes. Regular glucose monitoring and a balanced diet are crucial preventive measures.

2. **Weight Management:**

a. **Metabolic Slowdown:** The natural slowing of metabolism post-menopause may lead to weight gain. Adopting a healthy diet and engaging in regular physical activity are vital for weight management and overall well-being.

Mental Health

1. **Cognitive Decline:**

a. **Hormonal Influence:** Estrogen has a neuroprotective effect, and its decline post-menopause may contribute to cognitive decline. Mental stimulation, a balanced diet, and staying socially active support cognitive health.

2. **Mood Disorders:**

a. **Increased Vulnerability:** Post-menopausal women may be more vulnerable to mood disorders, including depression and anxiety. Regular mental health check-ups, counseling, and support networks play crucial roles in mental well-being.

Genitourinary Health

1. **Vaginal Atrophy:**

Estrogen's Impact: The decline in estrogen levels post-menopause can lead to vaginal atrophy, causing dryness, discomfort, and an increased risk of infections. Hormone therapy or alternative treatments can address these concerns.

2. **Urinary Incontinence:**

a. **Connectivity to Hormonal Changes:** Hormonal shifts post-menopause may contribute to urinary incontinence. Pelvic floor exercises and medical interventions can help manage this issue.

Breast Health:

1. **Breast Cancer Risk:**

a. **Ongoing Surveillance:** Post-menopausal women remain at risk for breast cancer. Regular mammograms, self-examinations, and consultations with healthcare providers are critical for early detection and management.

Sexual Health:

1. **Decreased Libido:**

a. **Hormonal Influence:** Hormonal changes post-menopause may lead to a decline in libido. Open communication with partners and healthcare providers can address concerns and explore potential solutions.

2. **Vaginal Dryness:**

a. **Impact on Intimacy:** Vaginal dryness can affect sexual comfort. Lubricants, hormone therapy, and candid discussions with healthcare providers contribute to a positive sexual experience.

Joint and Muscle Health

1. **Musculoskeletal Changes:**

a. **Estrogen's Role:** Estrogen's decline can contribute to joint and muscle discomfort. Regular exercise, including strength training, and a balanced diet support musculoskeletal health.

Vision Health

1. **Increased Risk of Eye Conditions:**

a. **Connectivity to Hormones:** Hormonal changes post-menopause may contribute to an increased risk of eye conditions such as dry eyes and macular degeneration. Regular eye check-ups are essential for preventive care.

Gastrointestinal Health

1. **Changes in Digestive Function:**

a. **Hormonal Impact:** Hormonal fluctuations can influence digestive function post-menopause. A fiber-rich diet, hydration, and regular gastrointestinal check-ups contribute to digestive health.

Skin Health
1. **Collagen Loss:**
a. **Estrogen's Influence:** Collagen loss, influenced by estrogen decline, can lead to changes in skin elasticity. Adequate hydration, sun protection, and skincare routines support skin health.

Overall Cancer Risks
1. **Endometrial and Ovarian Cancers:**
a. **Hormonal Factors:** Post-menopausal women may still be at risk for certain cancers. Regular screenings, including Pap smears and pelvic exams, are crucial for early detection and preventive care.

Importance Of Ongoing Health Monitoring

As women transition through this period, the importance of ongoing health monitoring cannot be overstated. This comprehensive and extensive note explores the critical significance of continuous health monitoring in post-menopause, emphasizing the multifaceted aspects that contribute to overall well-being.

1. **Hormonal Changes:** Menopause is characterized by a decline in estrogen and progesterone levels. Ongoing health monitoring allows healthcare professionals to assess and address the impact of these hormonal changes on various aspects of health, including bone density, cardiovascular health, and reproductive health.

2. **Bone Health:** Postmenopausal women are at an increased risk of osteoporosis due to the decline in estrogen levels. Regular monitoring through bone density scans helps in identifying bone loss early, allowing for interventions such as calcium supplementation, vitamin D, and weight-bearing exercises to maintain bone health.

3. **Cardiovascular Health:** Menopausal hormonal changes can influence cardiovascular health, potentially increasing the risk of heart disease. Ongoing monitoring of blood pressure, cholesterol levels, and other cardiovascular markers aids in the early detection of any issues, facilitating timely interventions and lifestyle modifications.

4. **Gynecological Screenings:** Regular gynecological screenings, including Pap smears and mammograms, are crucial during menopause to monitor for signs of gynecological cancers. Early detection enhances the effectiveness of treatment and improves overall outcomes.

5. **Pelvic Health:** Menopausal women may experience changes in pelvic health, including alterations in vaginal tissue and an increased risk of urinary incontinence. Monitoring and discussing these changes with healthcare providers allow for appropriate interventions and management strategies.

6. **Mental Health:** Hormonal fluctuations during menopause can impact mental health, contributing to mood swings and an increased risk of depression or anxiety. Ongoing monitoring allows for the identification of mental health concerns, facilitating timely intervention, and providing necessary support.

7. **Metabolic Health:** Menopausal hormonal changes may affect metabolism and body composition, potentially leading to weight gain and changes in lipid profiles. Regular monitoring of metabolic markers helps in the early identification of issues, allowing for lifestyle modifications and targeted interventions.

8. **Blood Sugar Levels:** The risk of developing insulin resistance and type 2 diabetes may increase during menopause. Monitoring blood sugar levels helps in the early detection of diabetes-related issues, enabling lifestyle modifications and, if necessary, medical interventions.

9. **Sexual Health:** Changes in sexual health, such as vaginal dryness and discomfort, are common during menopause. Ongoing monitoring and open communication with healthcare providers allow for the discussion of sexual health concerns, leading to appropriate interventions and the enhancement of overall well-being.

10. **Hormone Replacement Therapy (HRT):** For women considering or undergoing hormone replacement therapy (HRT), ongoing monitoring is crucial. Regular assessments of hormone levels and potential side effects allow for adjustments in treatment plans to ensure optimal benefits and minimize risks.

11. **Lifestyle Modifications:** Ongoing health monitoring provides an opportunity to assess the impact of lifestyle choices on menopausal symptoms and overall health. Healthcare providers can offer guidance on diet, exercise, stress management, and other lifestyle modifications to promote well-being.

12. **Individualized Care:** Menopausal experiences vary among women, and ongoing health monitoring allows for individualized care plans. Regular check-ups provide opportunities for women to discuss their unique symptoms, concerns, and preferences with healthcare providers, fostering a collaborative and tailored approach to healthcare.

CHAPTER NINE

WOMEN'S MENTAL HEALTH DURING AND AFTER MENOPAUSE

Hormonal Influences On Mood

Menopause, a natural biological process marking the end of a woman's reproductive years, is characterized by the cessation of menstrual cycles. This transitional phase is accompanied by significant hormonal fluctuations, particularly a decline in estrogen and progesterone levels, which can exert profound influences on mood and emotional well-being. Understanding the intricate interplay between hormones and mood during and after menopause is crucial for comprehending the challenges women may face in this stage of life.

1.　　Hormonal Changes during Menopause:

- **Estrogen Decline:** The most notable hormonal change during menopause is the decline in estrogen levels. Estrogen plays a crucial role in regulating various physiological functions, including those related to mood and emotional stability. Reduced estrogen levels have been associated with an increased risk of mood disturbances.

- **Progesterone Decline:** Progesterone, another important reproductive hormone, also declines during menopause. Although its direct impact on mood is not as extensively studied as estrogen, some research suggests that progesterone may have mood-stabilizing effects.

- **Impact on Neurotransmitters:** Estrogen has an intricate relationship with neurotransmitters like serotonin, dopamine, and norepinephrine, which play key roles in mood regulation. The decline in estrogen levels may disrupt the delicate balance of these neurotransmitters, potentially contributing to mood changes.

2.   Mood Changes during Menopause:

- **Mood Swings:** Fluctuating hormone levels can contribute to mood swings, characterized by sudden and intense changes in mood. Women may experience heightened irritability, frustration, or feelings of sadness.

- **Depression and Anxiety:** Some women may be more vulnerable to developing depression or anxiety during menopause. The hormonal shifts, coupled with life changes and societal factors, can contribute to the onset or exacerbation of these mood disorders.

- **Sleep Disturbances:** Hormonal changes can also affect sleep patterns, leading to insomnia or disrupted sleep. Sleep disturbances, in turn, can significantly impact mood and exacerbate feelings of irritability and fatigue.

3.   Postmenopausal Hormonal Influences:

- **Hormone Replacement Therapy (HRT):** Some women opt for hormone replacement therapy to alleviate menopausal symptoms, including mood disturbances. HRT involves supplementing estrogen and, in some cases, progesterone. The decision to undergo HRT should be made after careful consideration of potential risks and benefits.

- **Long-Term Impact:** Postmenopausal years may present a continued challenge for mood regulation. The absence of estrogen and progesterone, coupled with age-related changes in brain function, can contribute to a higher risk of mood disorders such as depression.

Coping Strategies For Emotional Well-Being

Alongside the physical symptoms, menopause can also bring about significant emotional challenges for many women. Coping with these changes is crucial for maintaining emotional well-being during and after this transitional phase.

1. **Educate Yourself:** Understanding the physiological and hormonal changes associated with menopause is the first step towards coping effectively. This

knowledge empowers women to anticipate and recognize the symptoms, reducing anxiety and uncertainty.

2. **Open Communication:** Discussing menopause with friends, family, or a healthcare professional fosters a supportive environment. Sharing experiences and concerns can provide emotional relief and help women realize they are not alone in their journey.

3. **Healthy Lifestyle Choices:** Adopting a healthy lifestyle can significantly impact emotional well-being. Regular exercise, a balanced diet, and adequate sleep contribute to overall physical and mental health, helping to alleviate mood swings and fatigue associated with menopause.

4. **Mindfulness and Relaxation Techniques:** Practices such as meditation, deep breathing exercises, and yoga can help manage stress and anxiety. Mindfulness techniques promote emotional balance by encouraging a present-focused and non-judgmental awareness of one's thoughts and feelings.

5. **Hormone Replacement Therapy (HRT):** For some women, hormone replacement therapy may be a viable option to manage severe menopausal symptoms. However, it is crucial to consult with a healthcare professional to assess the potential risks and benefits based on individual health history.

6. **Counseling and Support Groups:** Seeking professional counseling or joining support groups can provide a safe space for women to express their feelings and receive guidance. Mental health professionals can offer coping strategies tailored to individual needs.

7. **Developing a Positive Mindset:** Embracing a positive mindset and viewing menopause as a natural phase of life can contribute to emotional well-being. Recognizing the opportunities for personal growth and self-discovery during this time can be empowering.

8. **Hobbies and Leisure Activities:** Engaging in activities that bring joy and fulfillment can act as a distraction from menopausal symptoms. Hobbies and leisure pursuits provide a sense of purpose and accomplishment, boosting overall emotional well-being.

9. **Maintaining Social Connections:** Building and sustaining social connections is crucial during menopause. Spending time with friends and loved ones provides emotional support and a sense of belonging, which can positively impact mood and mental health.

10. **Professional Guidance on Nutrition and Supplements:** Consulting with a nutritionist or healthcare provider to ensure a well-balanced diet and considering supplements such as vitamin D

and calcium can contribute to overall health during and after menopause.

Support Systems And Resources

The transition through menopause can be challenging, and having a robust support system and access to appropriate resources is crucial for navigating this phase successfullqy.

1. **Healthcare Professionals:** Access to knowledgeable and empathetic healthcare professionals is fundamental during menopause. Gynecologists, endocrinologists, and general practitioners can provide guidance, conduct relevant screenings, and offer evidence-based interventions to manage menopausal symptoms effectively.

2. **Educational Resources:** Comprehensive and accessible educational resources contribute to informed decision-making during menopause. Reliable websites, books, and pamphlets provide information about the physiological changes, symptom management, and available treatment options, empowering women to actively participate in their healthcare journey.

3. **Support Groups:** Joining menopause support groups, whether in-person or online, creates a sense of community and understanding. Sharing

experiences, concerns, and coping strategies with other women navigating similar challenges fosters emotional support and helps combat feelings of isolation.

4. **Mental Health Professionals:** Menopause can have a significant impact on mental health. Psychologists, counselors, or therapists specializing in women's health can offer emotional support, coping strategies, and mental health interventions to address concerns such as mood swings, anxiety, or depression.

5. **Women's Health Organizations:** Organizations dedicated to women's health, such as the North American Menopause Society (NAMS) or the International Menopause Society (IMS), provide valuable resources, guidelines, and expert insights. These organizations contribute to the dissemination of evidence-based information and promote awareness about menopause-related issues.

6. **Family and Friends:** Establishing open communication with family and friends is crucial. A supportive network can provide understanding, empathy, and practical assistance. Discussing menopausal experiences with loved ones fosters a supportive environment and strengthens interpersonal relationships.

7. **Holistic Healthcare Approaches:** Exploring holistic healthcare approaches, such as integrative medicine, acupuncture, or naturopathy, can complement conventional treatments. Many women find relief from symptoms through a combination of traditional and complementary therapies tailored to their individual needs.

8. **Dietary and Nutritional Guidance:** Nutritionists or dietitians specializing in women's health can offer guidance on dietary changes that may alleviate menopausal symptoms. A balanced diet rich in vitamins, minerals, and phytoestrogens can positively impact overall health during menopause.

9. **Physical Activity and Fitness Resources:** Engaging in regular physical activity is beneficial for managing menopausal symptoms. Accessing resources such as fitness classes, online workouts, or guidance from fitness professionals helps women incorporate appropriate exercises into their routine to support cardiovascular health and bone density.

10. **Employer Support:** A supportive workplace environment is essential during menopause. Employers can implement policies that acknowledge and accommodate menopausal symptoms, fostering understanding and flexibility. Employee assistance programs may offer resources

for managing work-related stress and health concerns.

11. **Government and Public Health Initiatives**: Government initiatives and public health campaigns can contribute to raising awareness about menopause. Efforts to destigmatize discussions around menopause, promote healthcare access, and ensure workplace accommodations enhance societal support for women going through this life stage.

12. **Online Platforms and Apps:** Utilizing online platforms and mobile apps dedicated to women's health can provide valuable tools for tracking symptoms, accessing information, and connecting with communities. Technology facilitates convenient access to resources that support women in managing their menopausal journey.

Cognitive Behavioral Therapy (CBT) For Menopausal Women

Cognitive Behavioral Therapy (CBT) is a widely recognized and effective therapeutic approach that focuses on the relationship between thoughts, feelings, and behaviors. While traditionally used for various mental health conditions, CBT has shown promising results in addressing the psychological symptoms associated with menopause. This comprehensive overview explores the principles, techniques, and benefits of CBT for menopausal women.

Understanding CBT

1.   **Principles of CBT:**
- CBT is rooted in the idea that our thoughts, feelings, and behaviors are interconnected.
- It aims to identify and modify negative thought patterns to promote positive behavioral changes and improve emotional well-being.

2.   **Collaborative and Goal-Oriented:**
- CBT is a collaborative process between the therapist and the individual.
- It is goal-oriented, focusing on specific, measurable objectives to address symptoms and improve overall functioning.

CBT for Menopausal Symptoms

1.   **Addressing Mood Swings and Emotional Instability:**
- Menopausal women often experience mood swings and emotional instability due to hormonal fluctuations.

- CBT helps individuals identify and challenge negative thought patterns contributing to mood disturbances.

2. **Managing Anxiety and Stress:**
- Anxiety and stress are common during menopause, impacting both mental and physical well-being.
- CBT equips women with coping strategies to manage stressors, altering thought processes that contribute to heightened anxiety.

3. **Coping with Sleep Disturbances:**
- Sleep disturbances are prevalent in menopausal women and can significantly impact daily functioning.
- CBT techniques, such as sleep hygiene and cognitive restructuring, can address the underlying thoughts contributing to insomnia.

CBT Techniques for Menopausal Women

1. **Cognitive Restructuring:**
- Identifying and challenging negative thought patterns related to menopausal symptoms.
- Replacing irrational thoughts with more balanced and realistic perspectives.

2. **Behavioral Activation:**
- Encouraging individuals to engage in positive activities that bring a sense of accomplishment and pleasure.

- Countering the tendency to withdraw from activities due to menopausal symptoms.

3.   **Mindfulness and Relaxation Techniques:**
- Incorporating mindfulness practices to increase awareness of the present moment.
- Teaching relaxation techniques, such as deep breathing and progressive muscle relaxation, to manage stress and anxiety.

Benefits of CBT for Menopausal Women

1.   **Symptom Reduction:**
- CBT has been shown to reduce the severity of menopausal symptoms, including mood disturbances and anxiety.
- The skills learned in therapy can be applied in daily life to manage symptoms effectively.

2.   **Improved Quality of Life:**
- By addressing the cognitive and behavioral aspects of menopausal challenges, CBT contributes to an overall improvement in the quality of life.
- Enhanced coping mechanisms positively impact daily functioning and interpersonal relationships.

3.   **Long-Term Coping Skills:**
- CBT equips menopausal women with long-term coping skills that extend beyond the therapy sessions.

- The acquired tools empower individuals to navigate future challenges and life transitions.

Integration with Medical Treatment:

1. **Collaboration with Healthcare Professionals:**
- CBT can be integrated with medical treatments, including hormone replacement therapy (HRT), to provide a holistic approach.
- Collaborative efforts between mental health professionals and healthcare providers enhance overall care for menopausal women.
2. **Personalized Treatment Plans:**
- Tailoring CBT interventions to the individual's unique needs ensures a personalized and effective treatment plan.
- Adjustments can be made to address evolving symptoms and goals throughout the menopausal transition.

Mindfulness And Stress Reduction Techniques

Menopause is a natural and transformative phase in a woman's life, marked by hormonal changes that can impact physical and mental well-being. Stress, often exacerbated by the symptoms of menopause, plays a significant role in the overall experience. Mindfulness and stress reduction techniques offer holistic approaches to managing the challenges associated with this life transition. This comprehensive exploration delves into the principles, techniques, and benefits of incorporating mindfulness practices into the lives of menopausal women.

1. **Understanding Mindfulness:** Mindfulness involves cultivating present-moment awareness without judgment. It encourages individuals to engage fully in the current experience, acknowledging thoughts and feelings without becoming overwhelmed by them.

2. **Mindful Breathing:** One fundamental mindfulness technique is mindful breathing. By focusing attention on the breath, individuals develop a heightened awareness of each inhalation and exhalation. This simple yet powerful practice can help manage stress, promoting a sense of calm and centeredness.

3. **Body Scan Meditation:** Body scan meditation involves systematically directing attention to different parts of the body, noting sensations without attachment or judgment. This practice

enhances body awareness and can be effective in releasing tension and promoting relaxation.

4. **Mindful Walking:** Mindful walking encourages individuals to pay attention to each step, the sensation of movement, and the surrounding environment. This practice fosters a sense of grounding and can be particularly beneficial for managing stress-related symptoms.

5. **Guided Imagery:** Guided imagery involves visualizing calming and positive scenes. It allows individuals to create a mental sanctuary, providing an escape from stressors. Guided imagery can be a valuable tool in managing anxiety and promoting emotional well-being.

6. **Mindful Eating:** Mindful eating involves savoring each bite, paying attention to taste, texture, and the act of eating itself. By fostering a conscious relationship with food, individuals can reduce stress-related emotional eating and promote healthier dietary habits.

7. **Mindfulness-Based Stress Reduction (MBSR):** MBSR, a structured program developed by Dr. Jon Kabat-Zinn, integrates mindfulness meditation and yoga. It has been widely studied and found

effective in reducing stress, anxiety, and improving overall mental well-being.

8. **Acceptance and Commitment Therapy (ACT):** ACT, a mindfulness-based therapeutic approach, encourages individuals to accept their thoughts and feelings while committing to actions aligned with their values. This can be particularly empowering during the emotional fluctuations of menopause.

9. **Mindfulness Apps and Resources:** The digital age has brought forth a plethora of mindfulness apps and online resources. Platforms like Headspace, Calm, and Insight Timer offer guided meditations, breathing exercises, and mindfulness practices tailored to individual preferences and schedules.

10. **Mindfulness in Daily Activities:** Integrating mindfulness into daily activities, such as washing dishes or walking, transforms routine tasks into opportunities for presence and awareness. This approach promotes a mindful lifestyle, fostering resilience in the face of stressors.

11. **Yoga and Mindful Movement:** Yoga combines physical postures with breath awareness, promoting flexibility and relaxation. Mindful

movement practices like tai chi and qigong also enhance body-mind connection, providing stress-reducing benefits during menopause.

12. **Mindfulness-Based Cognitive Therapy (MBCT):** MBCT, an adaptation of CBT, combines mindfulness practices with cognitive therapy. It has shown efficacy in preventing the recurrence of depressive symptoms and may be beneficial for women experiencing mood changes during menopause.

CHAPTER ELEVEN

MAINTAINING BONE HEALTH POST-MENOPAUSE

Osteoporosis Risk Factors

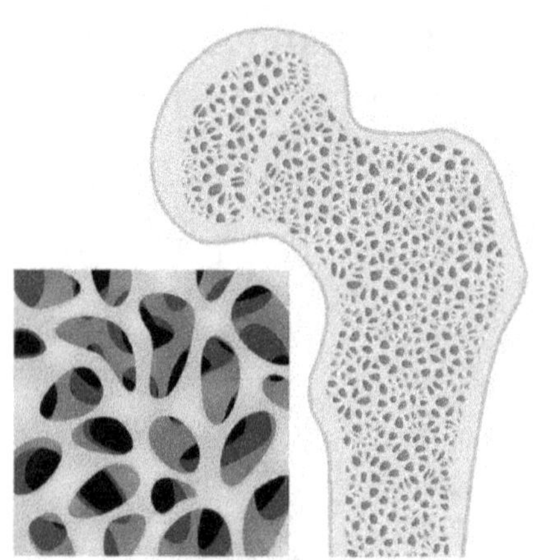

Healthy bone

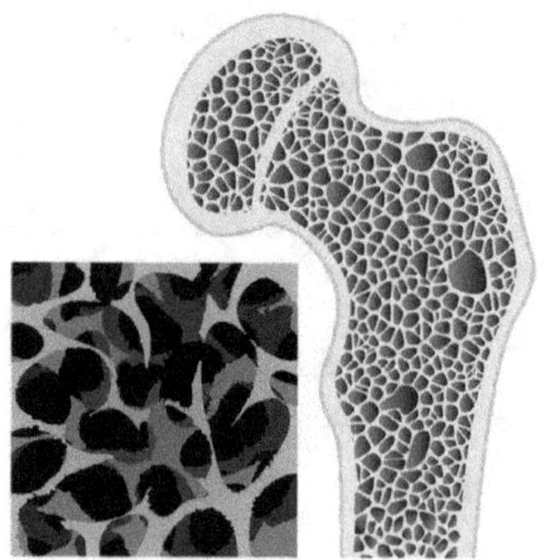

Osteoporosis

Osteoporosis is a common skeletal disorder characterized by low bone mass and deterioration of bone tissue, leading to an increased risk of fractures. Post-menopausal women are particularly susceptible to osteoporosis due to hormonal changes that affect bone density. This in-depth analysis explores the risk factors associated with osteoporosis in post-menopausal women, emphasizing the crucial relationship between these factors and bone health.

I.   Hormonal Changes and Bone Density

Estrogen Deficiency:
- Estrogen plays a pivotal role in maintaining bone density by inhibiting bone resorption.
- During menopause, there is a significant decline in estrogen levels, leading to increased bone turnover and decreased bone mineral density (BMD).

Accelerated Bone Loss:
- In the initial years of menopause, women may experience accelerated bone loss, particularly in the trabecular bone of the spine and hip.
- The rapid decline in estrogen contributes to increased osteoclast activity, leading to bone resorption.

II.   Age as a Risk Factor:

Post-Menopausal Age:
- Aging is an independent risk factor for osteoporosis.
- Post-menopausal women, especially those over 50, face an increased risk as bone resorption surpasses bone formation.

Bone Remodeling Imbalance:
- With age, the balance between bone formation and resorption shifts, favoring bone loss.

- Reduced bone density and compromised bone microarchitecture increase the susceptibility to fractures.

III.   Lifestyle Factors:

Nutritional Deficiencies:
- Inadequate calcium and vitamin D intake contributes to diminished bone density.
- Post-menopausal women should ensure sufficient dietary intake of these nutrients or consider supplementation.

Physical Inactivity:
- Lack of weight-bearing exercises diminishes bone density.
- Regular physical activity, especially weight-bearing and resistance exercises, helps maintain bone strength and reduce the risk of fractures.

IV.   Body Composition and Genetics:

Low Body Weight:
- Women with a lower body weight may have lower bone mass, increasing the risk of osteoporosis.
- Maintaining a healthy body weight through proper nutrition is crucial for bone health.

Genetic Factors:

- Family history of osteoporosis increases the risk, indicating a genetic predisposition.
- Genetic factors influence peak bone mass and the rate of bone loss during menopause.

V.   Other Medical Conditions and Medications:

Endocrine Disorders:
- Conditions such as hyperthyroidism and hyperparathyroidism can affect bone metabolism and increase the risk of osteoporosis.
- Management of underlying endocrine disorders is crucial for preserving bone health.

Medications:
- Prolonged use of certain medications, such as glucocorticoids, can lead to bone loss.
- Post-menopausal women on such medications should be monitored closely, and preventive measures should be considered.

VI.   Personal Habits and Lifestyle Choices:

Smoking:
- Smoking is associated with decreased bone density and an increased risk of fractures.
- Smoking cessation is beneficial for overall health, including bone health.

Excessive Alcohol Consumption:

- Heavy alcohol consumption negatively impacts bone health.
- Limiting alcohol intake is essential for minimizing the risk of osteoporosis
.

VII.   Screening and Prevention:

Bone Density Testing:
- Dual-energy X-ray absorptiometry (DXA) is the gold standard for assessing bone density.
- Post-menopausal women, especially those with risk factors, should undergo regular bone density testing.

Preventive Measures:
- Calcium and vitamin D supplementation may be recommended to meet nutritional needs.
- Lifestyle modifications, including weight-bearing exercises and a balanced diet, are crucial for preventing osteoporosis.

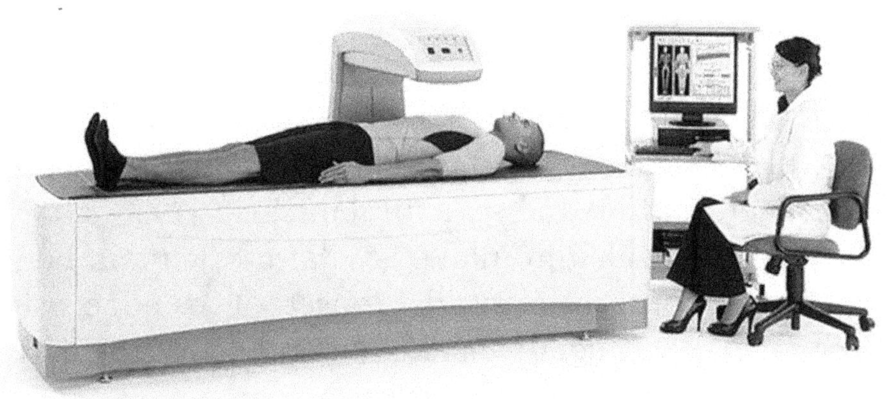

Dual-energy X-ray absorptiometry (DXA)

Importance Of Calcium And Vitamin d Intake

Post-menopause marks a critical phase in a woman's life, characterized by hormonal changes that can significantly impact bone health. Adequate intake of calcium and vitamin D becomes paramount during this period to mitigate the risk of osteoporosis and maintain overall well-being. This comprehensive exploration delves into the importance of calcium and vitamin D for post-menopausal women, outlining their roles, dietary sources, recommended intake, and the implications of deficiency.

I.   Role of Calcium in Post-Menopausal Bone Health:

Bone Mineralization:
- Calcium is a crucial mineral essential for bone mineralization and structural integrity.
- Adequate calcium intake is vital to maintain bone density and prevent the onset of osteoporosis, which post-menopausal women are particularly susceptible to due to hormonal changes.

Calcium Absorption and Hormonal Changes:
- Post-menopause, estrogen levels decline, affecting calcium absorption.
- Supplementation becomes crucial to meet calcium needs as hormonal changes can compromise the body's ability to absorb this mineral efficiently.

II.   Vitamin D's Contribution to Bone Health:

Calcium Absorption Facilitation:
- Vitamin D plays a pivotal role in enhancing the absorption of calcium in the intestines.
- Post-menopausal women with reduced estrogen levels may benefit significantly from sufficient vitamin D to optimize calcium utilization.

Regulation of Bone Metabolism:
- Vitamin D contributes to bone health by regulating calcium and phosphorus metabolism.

- Adequate vitamin D levels help maintain a balance between bone formation and resorption, reducing the risk of fractures.

III. Recommended Daily Intake:

Calcium Intake Guidelines:
- Post-menopausal women are generally advised to consume 1,200 to 1,500 milligrams of calcium daily.
- Dietary sources include dairy products, leafy green vegetables, fortified foods, and supplements when necessary.

Vitamin D Intake Guidelines:
- Recommended vitamin D intake for post-menopausal women is often around 600 to 800 IU (International Units) per day.
- Sun exposure, dietary sources like fatty fish and fortified products, and supplements contribute to meeting vitamin D requirements.

IV. Dietary Sources of Calcium and Vitamin D:

Calcium-Rich Foods:
- Dairy products such as milk, cheese, and yogurt are excellent sources of calcium.
- Leafy green vegetables, fortified plant-based milk alternatives, and nuts also contribute to dietary calcium intake.

Vitamin D-Rich Foods:

Fatty fish like salmon and mackerel are rich in vitamin D.

Fortified foods, including certain dairy products, cereals, and orange juice, are additional sources.

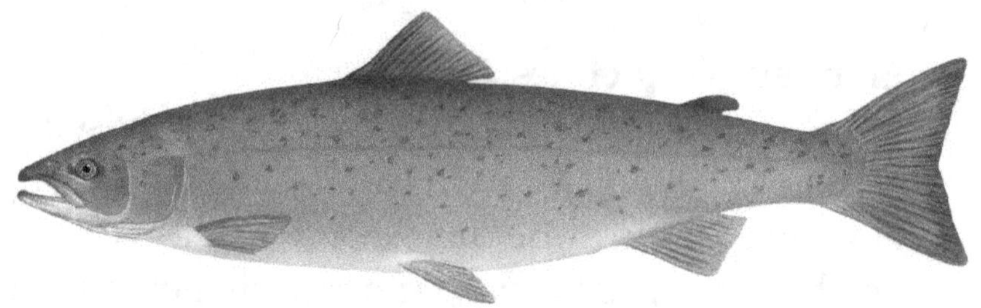

Salmon Fish

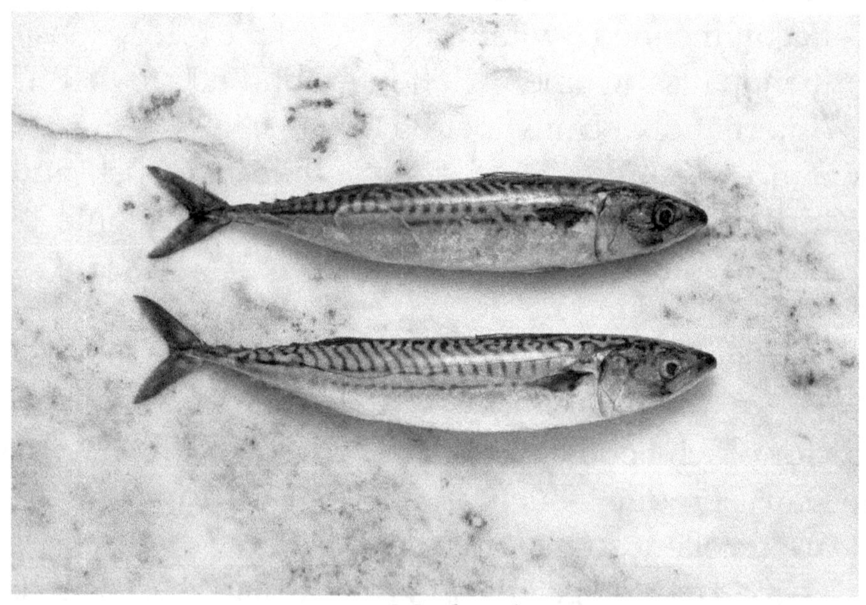

Mackerel

V.   Implications of Deficiency:

Osteoporosis Risk:

- Inadequate calcium and vitamin D intake increases the risk of osteoporosis, a condition characterized by weakened bones and an elevated susceptibility to fractures.

Muscle Weakness and Falls:

- Vitamin D deficiency is associated with muscle weakness, increasing the likelihood of falls and fractures.
- Adequate vitamin D levels are crucial for maintaining muscle function and balance.

VI.   Lifestyle Factors Affecting Absorption:

Sunlight Exposure:

- Vitamin D is synthesized in the skin upon exposure to sunlight.
- Limited sunlight exposure, common in certain geographic regions or due to lifestyle choices, can contribute to vitamin D deficiency.

Alcohol and Caffeine Consumption:

- Excessive alcohol and caffeine intake may interfere with calcium absorption.
- Moderation in the consumption of these substances is advisable for optimal bone health.

VII.   Supplements and Medical Guidance:

Supplementation Considerations:

- Supplements may be recommended for post-menopausal women who struggle to meet calcium and vitamin D requirements through diet alone.
- Consultation with healthcare professionals is essential to determine individual needs and potential interactions with other medications.

Regular Monitoring:

- Periodic monitoring of calcium and vitamin D levels is advisable to ensure adequacy and adjust supplementation if necessary.
- Healthcare providers can guide personalized approaches based on individual health status.

Weight-Bearing Exercises For Bone Density

Weight-bearing exercises are crucial for maintaining and improving bone density, especially as individuals age. These exercises involve working against gravity while on your feet and contribute to bone health by stimulating bone formation and reducing the risk of osteoporosis-related fractures. This guide outlines various weight-bearing exercises that can be incorporated into a fitness routine to enhance bone density.

1. **Brisk Walking:** Engaging in brisk walking is a simple yet effective weight-bearing exercise. The repetitive impact on your feet stimulates bone density in the lower extremities, particularly in the hips and legs. Ensure you maintain an upright posture and wear supportive footwear.

2. **Running and Jogging:** Running and jogging are higher-impact weight-bearing exercises that provide substantial mechanical stress to bones. These activities, when done with proper form and on supportive surfaces, contribute significantly to bone density, especially in weight-bearing bones like the spine and legs.

3. **Aerobic Dancing:** Aerobic dance routines involve dynamic movements that engage multiple muscle groups, providing both cardiovascular benefits and weight-bearing impact. The varied steps and jumps in dance routines stimulate bone formation, particularly in the lower body.

4. **Jumping Rope:** Jumping rope is a high-impact exercise that places stress on the bones of the legs and hips. The repetitive nature of jumping contributes to bone density, and it also offers cardiovascular benefits. Ensure you use a proper surface and start at a comfortable pace.

5. **Stair Climbing:** Climbing stairs is a weight-bearing activity that targets the muscles and bones of the lower body. It provides a combination of resistance

and impact, making it effective for building bone density in the hips, thighs, and calves. Use proper handrail support if needed.

6. **Hiking:** Hiking involves walking on uneven terrain, adding an extra dimension to the mechanical stress on bones. The inclines and declines encountered during hiking engage various muscle groups and contribute to bone health, particularly in the legs and hips.

7. **Weightlifting:** Resistance training with weights, whether using free weights or machines, is a valuable weight-bearing exercise. Weightlifting engages the muscles and bones, promoting bone density and strengthening the skeletal structure. Focus on compound movements for comprehensive benefits.

8. **Body weight Exercises:** Incorporating body weight exercises like squats, lunges, and push-ups provides resistance to bones and muscles. These exercises engage multiple joints and muscle groups, promoting bone density in areas such as the spine, hips, and upper body.

9. **Resistance Band Workouts:** Utilizing resistance bands adds an element of resistance to various exercises. Resistance band workouts engage muscles and bones, promoting bone density. They offer a convenient and versatile option for resistance training.

10. **Functional Movements:** Engaging in functional movements that mimic activities of daily living, such as lifting, bending, and reaching, provides weight-bearing benefits. These movements stimulate bone formation while improving overall functional fitness.

CHAPTER TWELVE

CARDIOVASCULAR HEALTH IN POST-MENOPAUSE

Understanding Cardiovascular Risks

Post-menopause, a phase characterized by the cessation of menstrual cycles, introduces unique health considerations for women, particularly in the realm of cardiovascular health. This transition is accompanied by hormonal changes, primarily the decline in estrogen levels, which contributes to an increased vulnerability to cardiovascular diseases (CVD). Let's explore the cardiovascular risks in post-menopausal women, the underlying mechanisms, and strategies for prevention and management.

Cardiovascular Risks in Post-Menopause

Post-menopausal women face an elevated risk of heart disease compared to their pre-menopausal counterparts. The decline in estrogen levels, a hormone with protective effects on the cardiovascular system, is a key contributor to this increased vulnerability. Unfavorable changes in lipid profiles, such as an increase in low-density lipoprotein (LDL) cholesterol and a decrease in high-density lipoprotein

(HDL) cholesterol, further accentuate the cardiovascular risks.

Mechanisms Behind Cardiovascular Risks

The decline in estrogen post-menopause contributes to endothelial dysfunction, inflammation, and increased arterial stiffness. Metabolic changes, including an increase in visceral fat, may lead to insulin resistance and metabolic syndrome, elevating the risk of diabetes and subsequently contributing to cardiovascular risks. Blood pressure changes, characterized by increased arterial stiffness and alterations in vascular tone, also become more prevalent during this phase. Additionally, chronic inflammation, associated with an increase in inflammatory markers post-menopause, plays a role in the development and progression of atherosclerosis.

Cardiovascular Conditions Associated with Post-Menopause

1. Accelerated Atherosclerosis:

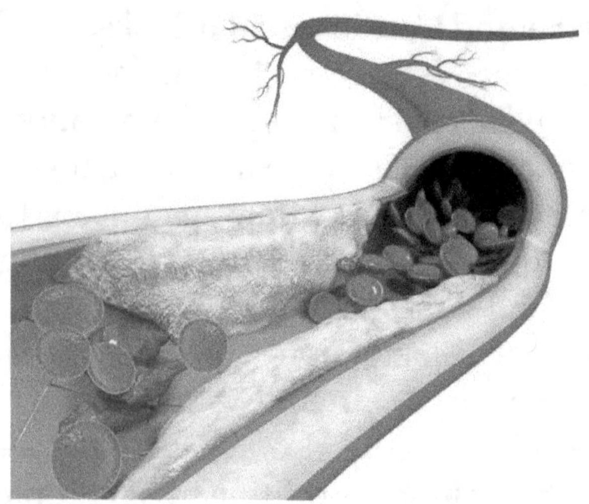

Post-menopausal women are prone to accelerated atherosclerosis, a condition characterized by the buildup of plaque in the arteries. The protective effects of estrogen on blood vessels diminish, leading to an increased risk of plaque formation and arterial narrowing.

2. Coronary Artery Disease (CAD):

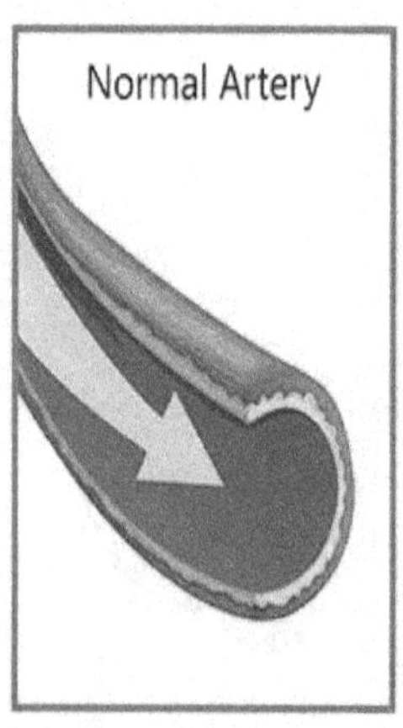

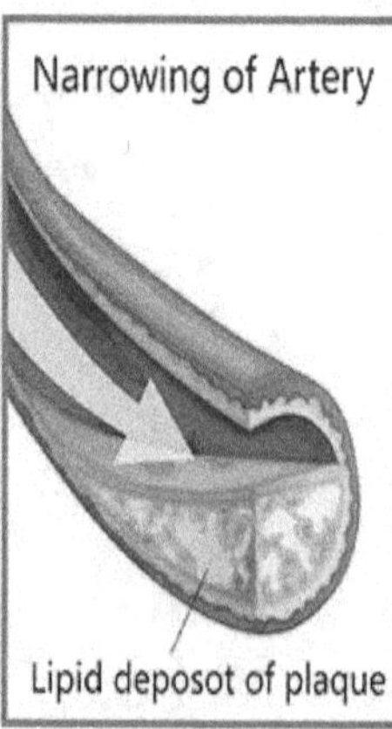

The decline in estrogen levels during post-menopause is associated with an elevated risk of coronary artery disease. This condition involves the narrowing of the coronary arteries, which supply blood to the heart muscle. Reduced estrogen contributes to coronary artery vasoconstriction, potentially leading to angina (chest pain) or, in severe cases, a heart attack.

3. Increased Risk of Hypertension:

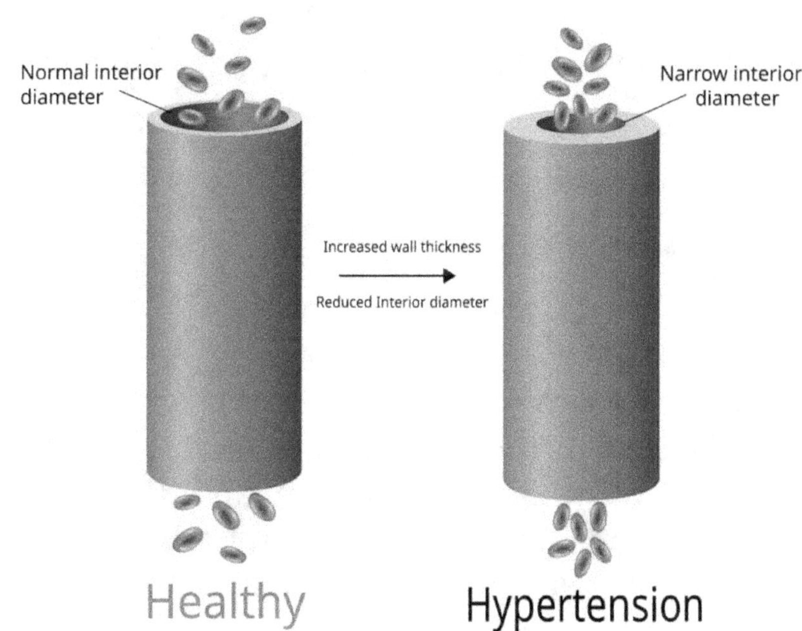

Post-menopausal women often experience alterations in blood pressure regulation. The hormonal changes and the aging process contribute to increased arterial stiffness, leading to hypertension. Hypertension is a significant risk factor for various cardiovascular complications, including stroke and heart failure.

4. Stroke Risk:

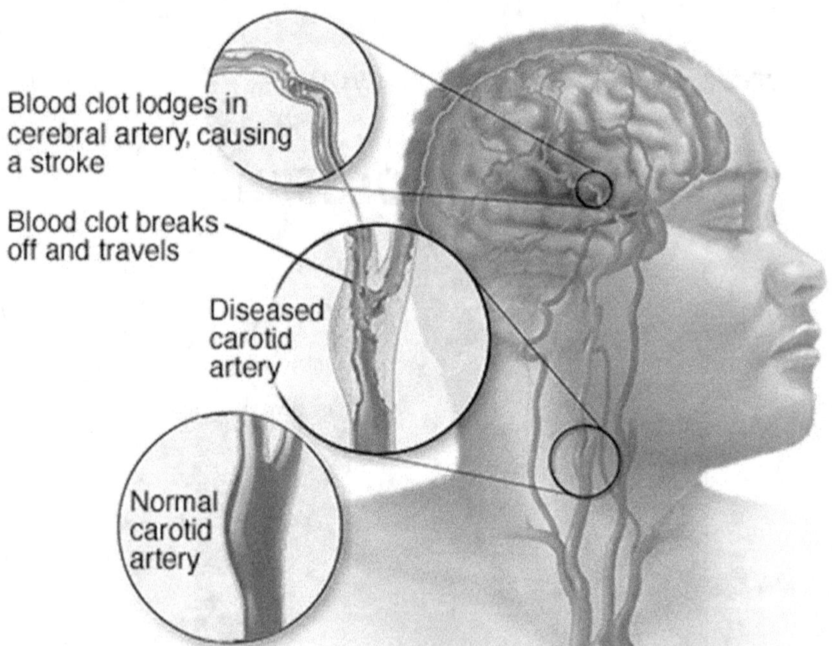

The decline in estrogen levels is associated with an increased risk of stroke in post-menopausal women. Changes in blood vessel function and the overall vascular environment contribute to this elevated risk. Stroke prevention strategies become crucial for maintaining cardiovascular health.

5. Heart Failure Risk:

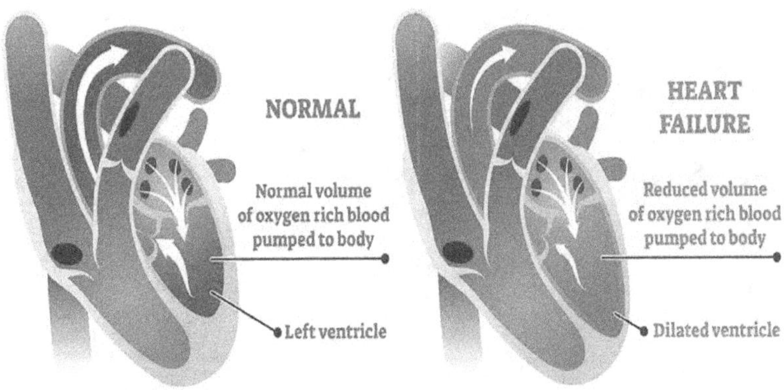

Post-menopausal women face an elevated risk of heart failure. The decline in estrogen is linked to changes in cardiac structure and function, making the heart more susceptible to impairment. Heart failure can result in symptoms such as shortness of breath, fatigue, and fluid retention.

6. Dyslipidemia:

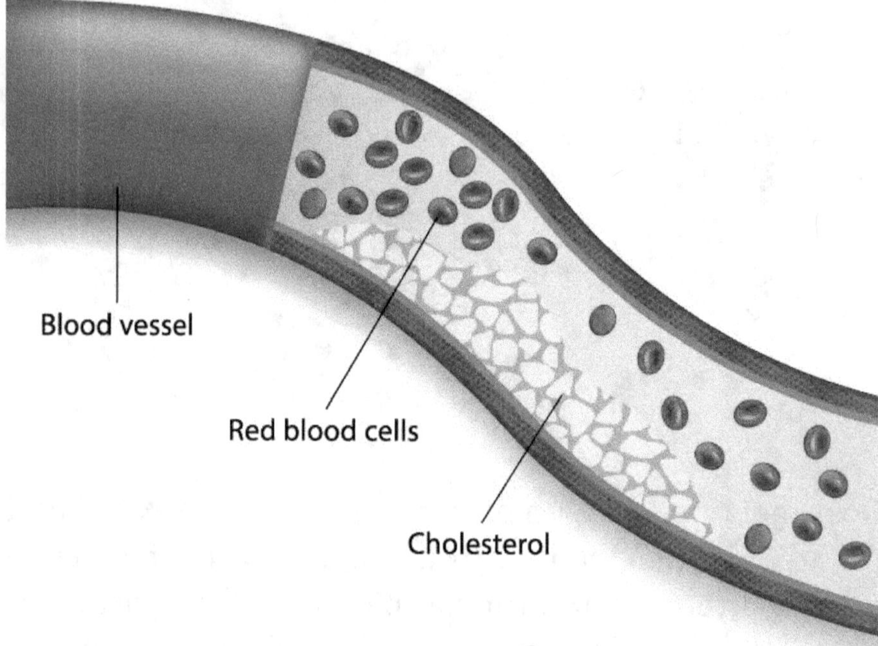

Menopause is accompanied by alterations in lipid profiles. There is often an increase in low-density lipoprotein (LDL) cholesterol and a decrease in high-density lipoprotein (HDL) cholesterol. Dyslipidemia is a significant contributor to atherosclerosis and cardiovascular events.

Endothelial Dysfunction:

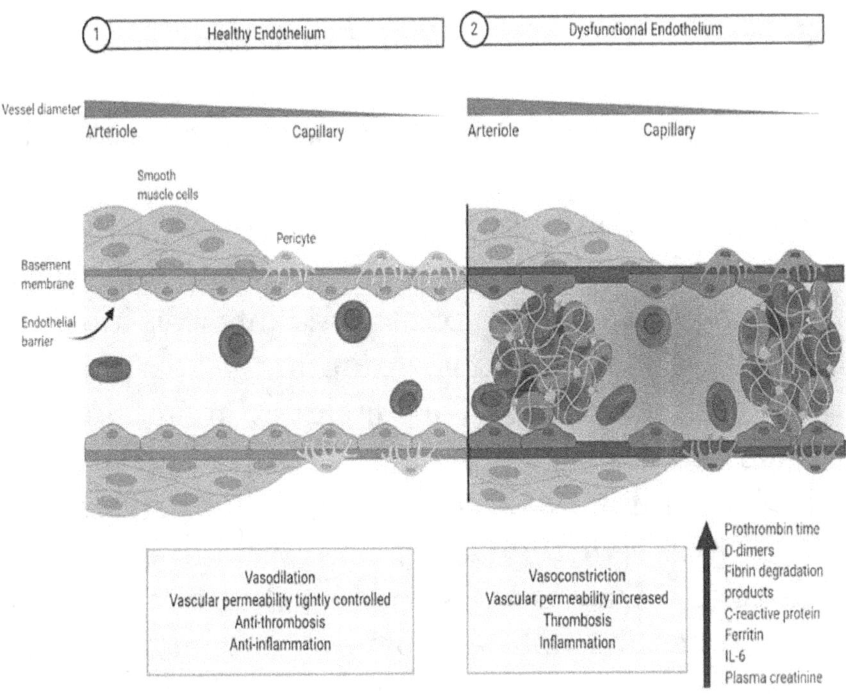

Estrogen plays a crucial role in maintaining the health of the endothelium, the inner lining of blood vessels. The decline in estrogen post-menopause contributes to endothelial dysfunction, impairing blood vessel function and promoting atherosclerosis.

Prevention and Management Strategies

1. **Hormone Replacement Therapy (HRT):** Hormone replacement therapy, involving the replacement of estrogen and, in some cases, progesterone, is a controversial but potentially beneficial option for managing cardiovascular risks in post-menopausal

women. However, its application requires careful consideration of individual health risks and benefits.

2. **Cardiovascular Risk Assessment:** Regular cardiovascular risk assessments, including lipid profiles, blood pressure monitoring, and an evaluation of other risk factors, are essential. Early identification allows for targeted interventions.

3. **Lifestyle Modifications:** Adopting a heart-healthy lifestyle is critical. This includes maintaining a balanced diet, engaging in regular physical activity, and avoiding tobacco use. Weight management and stress reduction also play pivotal roles.

4. **Regular Exercise:** Regular physical activity, encompassing both aerobic exercises and strength training, can help manage cardiovascular risks. Exercise contributes to weight management, improved lipid profiles, and enhanced cardiovascular function.

5. **Nutrition:** A heart-healthy diet, rich in fruits, vegetables, whole grains, and lean proteins, can help control cholesterol levels and blood pressure. Limiting saturated and trans fats, sodium, and added sugars is crucial.

6. **Blood Pressure Management:** Regular monitoring of blood pressure and appropriate management, which may include lifestyle changes and medications, is essential.

7. **Regular Health Check-ups:** Post-menopausal women should have regular check-ups with healthcare providers to monitor cardiovascular health. Timely interventions can help manage risk factors and prevent complications.

Lifestyle Changes For Heart Health

Post-menopause, the stage following the cessation of menstrual periods, is a critical time for women to focus on heart health. The decline in estrogen levels during menopause contributes to changes in cardiovascular risk factors, making it essential for women to adopt lifestyle changes that promote heart health. These changes encompass various aspects of daily living and contribute to overall well-being.

1. **Regular Physical Activity**: Engaging in regular exercise is pivotal for maintaining heart health during post-menopause. Aerobic exercises such as brisk walking, jogging, cycling, or swimming can help improve cardiovascular fitness, reduce blood pressure, and manage weight. Strength training is also beneficial for preserving muscle mass and supporting overall metabolism.
2. **Heart-Healthy Diet:** Adopting a heart-healthy diet is crucial for managing cardiovascular risk factors.

Post-menopausal women should focus on a balanced diet rich in fruits, vegetables, whole grains, lean proteins, and healthy fats. Limiting saturated and trans fats, cholesterol, and sodium helps control blood lipid levels and blood pressure.

3. **Omega-3 Fatty Acids:** Including sources of omega-3 fatty acids in the diet, such as fatty fish (e.g., salmon, mackerel), flaxseeds, chia seeds, and walnuts, can contribute to heart health. Omega-3 fatty acids have anti-inflammatory properties and may help reduce the risk of cardiovascular events.

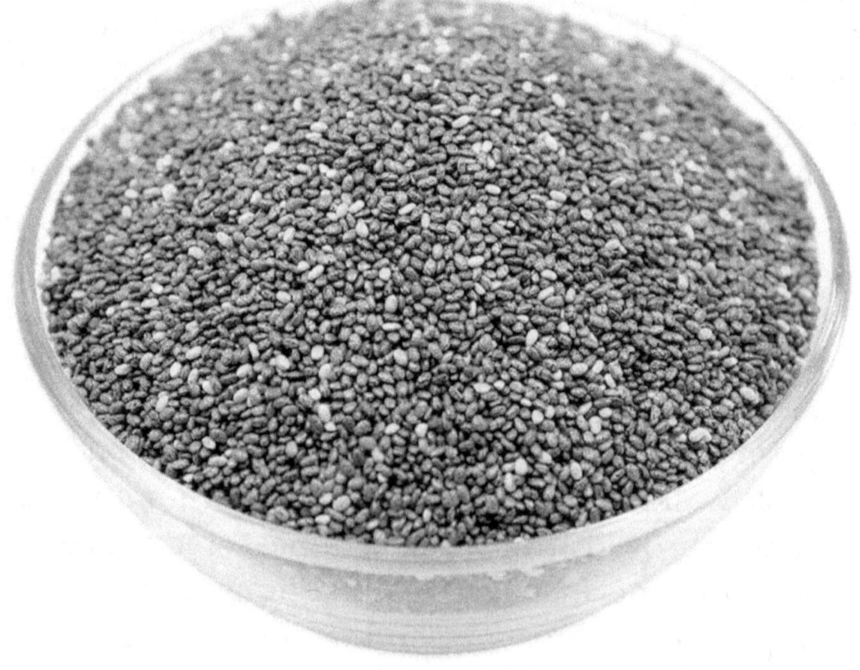

Chia seeds

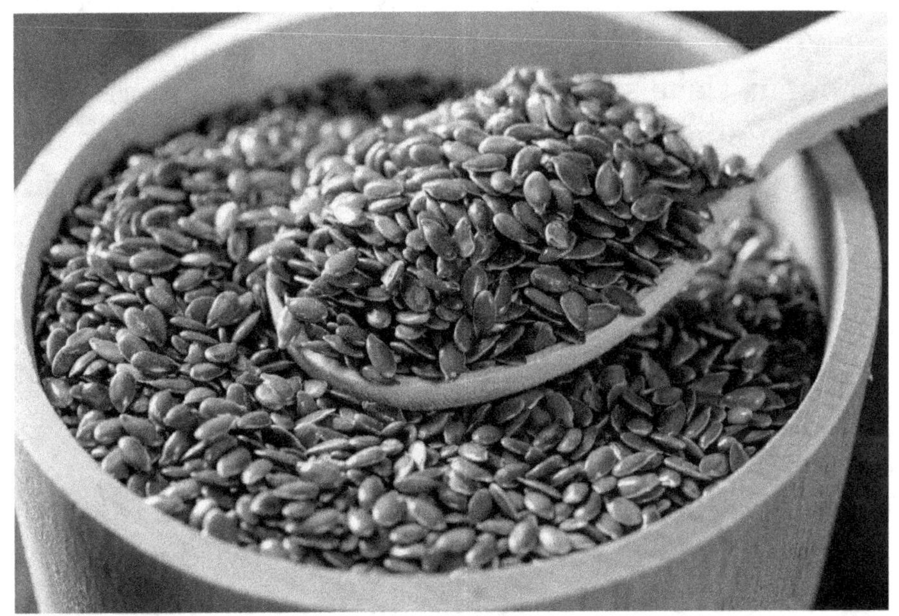

Flax seeds

4. **Maintain a Healthy Weight:** Post-menopausal women often experience changes in metabolism and an increased risk of weight gain. Maintaining a healthy weight through a combination of a balanced diet and regular exercise is crucial for preventing obesity, which is a significant risk factor for heart disease.

5. **Control Blood Pressure:** Monitoring and controlling blood pressure is essential for heart health. Lifestyle changes such as reducing sodium intake, maintaining a healthy weight, exercising regularly, and managing stress contribute to optimal blood pressure levels.

6. **Manage Blood Sugar Levels:** Post-menopausal women should be vigilant about managing blood sugar levels, especially if there is a risk of developing diabetes. A diet rich in fiber, regular physical activity, and weight management can contribute to stable blood sugar levels.

7. **Quit Smoking:** If applicable, quitting smoking is one of the most impactful lifestyle changes for heart health. Smoking is a significant risk factor for cardiovascular disease, and quitting improves overall cardiovascular well-being.

8. **Limit Alcohol Intake:** While moderate alcohol consumption may have some cardiovascular benefits, excessive alcohol intake can contribute to heart-related issues. Post-menopausal women should limit alcohol intake to moderate levels, which is generally defined as up to one drink per day for women.

9. **Manage Stress:** Chronic stress can negatively impact heart health. Adopting stress management techniques such as mindfulness, meditation, deep breathing exercises, or engaging in hobbies and activities that bring joy can contribute to emotional well-being and reduce the risk of heart disease.

10. **Adequate Sleep:** Quality sleep is essential for heart health. Post-menopausal women may experience sleep disturbances, and establishing good sleep hygiene practices, such as maintaining a consistent

sleep schedule, creating a comfortable sleep environment, and avoiding stimulants before bedtime, can contribute to better sleep quality.

11. **Regular Health Check-ups:** Regular health check-ups with healthcare professionals are crucial for monitoring cardiovascular risk factors. Blood lipid levels, blood pressure, and other relevant health markers should be routinely assessed. Healthcare providers can offer personalized advice based on individual health profiles.

12. **Stay Hydrated:** Adequate hydration is often overlooked but is essential for heart health. Staying well-hydrated supports overall cardiovascular function and helps maintain healthy blood flow.

Medications And Interventions

Managing cardiovascular health during post-menopause involves a multifaceted approach that may include medications and interventions tailored to individual risk factors and health conditions. This phase, marked by hormonal changes and an increased risk of cardiovascular disease, requires a comprehensive strategy to address potential challenges and optimize heart health.

Hormone Replacement Therapy (HRT): Hormone replacement therapy, specifically estrogen replacement, has been a subject of considerable discussion regarding its impact on cardiovascular health during post-menopause. While estrogen was once believed to have protective effects on the cardiovascular system, recent studies have raised concerns about its potential risks, particularly with long-term use. The decision to undergo HRT should be individualized, considering factors such as overall health, personal preferences, and potential risks and benefits.

Statins: Statins are a class of medications commonly prescribed to lower cholesterol levels. For post-menopausal women with elevated cholesterol levels, statins may be recommended to reduce the risk of atherosclerosis and cardiovascular events. These medications work by inhibiting the production of cholesterol in the liver and have demonstrated efficacy in managing lipid profiles.

Blood Pressure Medications: Hypertension is a significant cardiovascular risk factor, and post-menopausal women with high blood pressure may be prescribed antihypertensive medications. These medications, including ACE inhibitors, beta-blockers, diuretics, and calcium channel blockers, help lower blood pressure and reduce the workload on the heart, decreasing the risk of heart disease and stroke.

Antiplatelet Agents: Antiplatelet medications, such as aspirin, may be recommended for post-menopausal women with a history of cardiovascular events or those at high risk. These medications help prevent blood clot formation, reducing the likelihood of heart attacks and strokes. The decision to use antiplatelet therapy involves a careful assessment of individual risks and benefits.

Diabetes Medications: Post-menopausal women with diabetes may require medications to manage blood sugar levels effectively. Proper glycemic control is essential for preventing cardiovascular complications associated with diabetes. Medications such as metformin, sulfonylureas, or insulin may be prescribed based on individual needs.

Weight Management Medications: For post-menopausal women struggling with obesity, medications designed to aid weight management may be considered in conjunction with lifestyle modifications. These medications, such as orlistat or liraglutide, work by reducing calorie absorption or promoting feelings of fullness.

Angiotensin Receptor Blockers (ARBs): ARBs are another class of antihypertensive medications commonly prescribed to manage blood pressure. They block the effects of angiotensin II, a hormone that narrows blood vessels, helping to relax blood vessels and lower blood pressure. ARBs are often used when ACE inhibitors are not well-tolerated.

Nitroglycerin and Beta-Blockers for Angina: Women experiencing angina or chest pain due to reduced blood flow to the heart may be prescribed nitroglycerin or beta-blockers. Nitroglycerin helps relax and widen blood vessels, improving blood flow, while beta-blockers reduce the heart's workload and oxygen demand.

Cardiac Rehabilitation Programs: For women with a history of cardiovascular events or interventions, cardiac rehabilitation programs offer a comprehensive approach to recovery. These programs include supervised exercise, education on heart-healthy living, and support for psychological well-being.

Lifestyle Interventions: While medications play a crucial role, lifestyle interventions are integral to managing cardiovascular health during post-menopause. Adopting a heart-healthy diet, engaging in regular physical activity, managing stress, avoiding tobacco, and limiting alcohol intake contribute significantly to overall well-being.

Coronary Artery Bypass Grafting (CABG) and Angioplasty: In cases of severe coronary artery disease, interventions such as coronary artery bypass grafting (CABG) or angioplasty with stent placement may be recommended. These procedures aim to restore blood flow to the heart muscle and alleviate symptoms such as chest pain.

Continuous Monitoring and Follow-Up: Post-menopausal women with cardiovascular concerns require ongoing monitoring and regular follow-up with healthcare providers. This ensures that medications are optimized, interventions are effective, and any emerging health issues are promptly addressed.

CHAPTER THIRTEEN

WOMEN'S SEXUAL HEALTH IN POST-MENOPAUSE

Changes In Libido And Sexual Function

Post-menopause, a phase marking the end of the reproductive years, brings about a range of hormonal changes that can significantly influence libido and sexual function in women. Understanding these changes and addressing the associated challenges is crucial for promoting sexual well-being and maintaining healthy intimate relationships during this transformative life stage.

- **Hormonal Fluctuations:** The decline in estrogen and progesterone levels, hallmark hormonal changes during post-menopause, plays a central role in impacting sexual function. Estrogen, in particular, contributes to the health and elasticity of the vaginal tissues, and its reduction can lead to symptoms such as vaginal dryness and thinning.
- **Vaginal Dryness and Discomfort:** Reduced estrogen levels often result in vaginal dryness, causing discomfort during sexual activity. The lack of adequate lubrication can lead to irritation, pain,

and an overall decline in sexual satisfaction. Addressing vaginal dryness is a key aspect of managing sexual function post-menopause.

- **Changes in Sexual Desire:** Fluctuations in sexual desire are common during post-menopause. While some women experience a decrease in libido, others may find that their interest in sexual activity remains unchanged or may even increase. Individual variations in response highlight the complex interplay of hormonal, psychological, and interpersonal factors.

- **Psychological and Emotional Factors:** Emotional and psychological well-being significantly influences sexual function. Post-menopausal women may contend with stress, anxiety, or body image concerns, which can impact libido. Addressing these factors through open communication, emotional support, and, if necessary, professional counseling is essential.

- **Relationship Dynamics:** Changes in sexual function can affect intimate relationships. Communication with partners about these changes, understanding each other's needs, and fostering emotional intimacy are crucial for maintaining a healthy and satisfying sexual connection during post-menopause.

- **Self-Esteem and Body Image:** Shifts in sexual function can sometimes impact self-esteem and body image. Women may grapple with feelings of inadequacy or changes in how they perceive their own desirability. Cultivating positive self-image and self-acceptance becomes essential for overall well-being.

- **Pelvic Floor Changes:** Hormonal changes can contribute to alterations in the pelvic floor muscles, potentially affecting sexual function. Pelvic floor exercises, such as Kegel exercises, may be recommended to enhance pelvic floor tone and improve sexual satisfaction.

- **Medical Conditions and Medications:** Certain medical conditions, such as cardiovascular disease, diabetes, or arthritis, as well as medications used to manage these conditions, can influence sexual function. Consulting with healthcare providers about potential side effects and exploring alternative medications when possible is crucial.

- **Hormone Replacement Therapy (HRT):** Hormone replacement therapy, particularly local estrogen therapy, is a common intervention to address symptoms such as vaginal dryness and discomfort. HRT aims to replenish estrogen levels in the vaginal tissues, alleviating specific symptoms associated with post-menopausal changes.

- **Lubricants and Moisturizers:** Over-the-counter or prescription vaginal lubricants and moisturizers can provide relief from vaginal dryness. These products aim to enhance lubrication and maintain vaginal health, promoting comfort during sexual activity.

- **Sexual Wellness Therapies:** Professional sexual wellness therapies, such as sex therapy or counseling, offer valuable support for post-menopausal women experiencing challenges in their sexual lives. These therapeutic approaches focus on communication, education, and practical strategies to enhance sexual satisfaction.

- **Regular Gynecological Check-ups:** Regular gynecological check-ups are essential during post-menopause to monitor pelvic health and address any concerns related to sexual function. Gynecologists can offer guidance, recommend interventions, and provide support tailored to individual needs.

- **Alternative Therapies:** Some women explore alternative therapies, such as acupuncture or herbal supplements, to address sexual concerns. While the evidence for the effectiveness of these approaches varies, individual experiences and preferences should be considered.

Communication With Partners

Effective communication with partners during post-menopause is crucial for maintaining emotional intimacy, addressing changes in sexual dynamics, and navigating the various challenges that may arise during this life stage. Post-menopause, characterized by hormonal shifts and associated physical and emotional changes, can impact both individuals in a relationship. Open and empathetic communication fosters understanding, strengthens the relationship, and helps couples adapt to the evolving dynamics of this phase.

- **Honest and Open Dialogues:** Establishing a foundation of honest and open communication is essential. Encouraging an environment where both partners feel comfortable expressing their thoughts, concerns, and feelings sets the stage for productive discussions about post-menopausal experiences.
- **Educate and Share Information:** Post-menopause is often accompanied by a range of physical changes, including fluctuations in libido, vaginal dryness, and mood swings. Sharing information about these changes, either through discussions or by jointly researching reputable sources, helps both partners understand the biological aspects of post-menopause and reduces misconceptions.
- **Express Emotional Needs:** Emotional intimacy is as vital as physical intimacy in a relationship. Encourage each other to express emotional needs and provide support during times of vulnerability.

Creating a safe space for emotional sharing enhances the bond between partners.

- **Discuss Sexual Health:** Changes in sexual desire, arousal, and satisfaction may occur during post-menopause. Initiating a conversation about sexual health is essential. Discussing preferences, concerns, and exploring new ways to maintain intimacy can contribute to a fulfilling and satisfying sexual relationship.

- **Address Vaginal Dryness and Discomfort:** Vaginal dryness is a common symptom during post-menopause that can impact sexual comfort. Discussing this issue openly and considering solutions together, such as the use of lubricants or seeking medical advice, demonstrates mutual concern for each other's well-being.

- **Seek Professional Guidance:** If challenges persist, seeking the guidance of a healthcare professional or a sex therapist can be beneficial. These experts can provide specialized advice, offer solutions, and facilitate constructive conversations around sexual health.

- **Explore Intimacy Beyond Sex:** Intimacy extends beyond sexual activity. Engage in non-sexual forms of intimacy, such as cuddling, hugging, and verbal expressions of affection. Focusing on emotional connection strengthens the overall bond between partners.

- **Be Patient and Understanding:** Patience and understanding are crucial virtues during post-menopause. Both partners may be navigating uncharted territory, and empathy plays a pivotal role in fostering mutual support and cooperation.
- **Encourage Self-Care:** Encouraging self-care is an important aspect of communication. Both partners should prioritize self-care practices, including regular exercise, healthy nutrition, and stress management, which contribute to overall well-being and can positively impact the relationship.
- **Share Relationship Goals:** Discussing long-term relationship goals is vital. Establish shared expectations, explore mutual aspirations, and align on how to support each other through the various life stages that come with post-menopause.
- **Embrace Changes Together:** Change is inevitable, and post-menopause brings about significant changes. Embrace these changes together as a team. Collaborate on finding adaptive strategies, exploring new facets of the relationship, and celebrating the enduring bond that has been built over time.
- **Celebrate Intimacy Milestones:** Celebrate milestones in intimacy, no matter how small. Recognizing and appreciating positive experiences fosters a positive outlook and reinforces the idea that intimacy can evolve and deepen over time.

- **Stay Attuned to Emotional Cues:** Pay attention to emotional cues and non-verbal communication. Sometimes, partners may convey their feelings through subtle gestures or changes in behavior. Staying attuned to these cues enables a deeper understanding of each other's emotional states.

Therapeutic Options For Sexual Health

Therapeutic options for sexual health in post-menopause encompass a range of interventions designed to address the physical, emotional, and relational aspects of sexual well-being. The post-menopausal phase, characterized by hormonal changes, can present challenges in terms of libido, vaginal health, and overall sexual satisfaction. Understanding and exploring therapeutic options empower women to navigate this phase with enhanced sexual vitality and well-being.

- **Hormone Replacement Therapy (HRT):** Hormone replacement therapy, specifically local estrogen therapy, is a common therapeutic option for post-menopausal women experiencing vaginal dryness, discomfort, and atrophy. Estrogen creams, rings, or tablets can be applied directly to the vaginal tissues, promoting increased moisture, improved elasticity, and reduced discomfort during sexual activity.

- **Non-Hormonal Moisturizers and Lubricants:** Over-the-counter and prescription vaginal moisturizers and lubricants offer a non-hormonal approach to addressing vaginal dryness and discomfort. These products provide immediate relief during sexual activity and can be used regularly to maintain vaginal health.
- **Pelvic Floor Physical Therapy:** Pelvic floor physical therapy focuses on exercises and techniques to strengthen and improve the flexibility of pelvic floor muscles. This therapy can enhance sexual function by addressing issues such as pelvic pain, muscle tension, and urinary incontinence.
- **Sexual Wellness Counseling or Therapy:** Seeking the guidance of a sex therapist or counselor specializing in sexual wellness can be beneficial for post-menopausal women facing challenges in their sexual lives. These professionals offer a safe space to discuss concerns, explore communication strategies with partners, and provide education on sexual health.
- **Couples Therapy:** Couples therapy can be valuable for addressing relational dynamics and enhancing communication between partners. Post-menopausal women and their partners can work together to navigate changes in sexual desire,

explore new ways of intimacy, and foster emotional connection.

- **Educational Programs:** Participating in educational programs focused on sexual health during menopause can provide valuable information and resources. Workshops, seminars, or online courses led by healthcare professionals or sex educators offer insights into managing changes and maintaining a satisfying sexual life.
- **Alternative Therapies:** Some women explore alternative therapies, such as acupuncture or mindfulness practices, to promote relaxation, reduce stress, and enhance overall well-being. While the evidence for the efficacy of these approaches in sexual health is varied, individual preferences and experiences should be considered.
- **Phosphodiesterase Type 5 (PDE5) Inhibitors:** PDE5 inhibitors, commonly used to treat erectile dysfunction in men, have shown promise in improving sexual function for post-menopausal women. Medications such as sildenafil or tadalafil may enhance blood flow to the genital area, potentially improving arousal and satisfaction.
- **Testosterone Replacement Therapy:** Testosterone, though primarily associated with male hormones, also plays a role in female sexual function. Some post-menopausal women may benefit from testosterone replacement therapy to address

concerns related to low libido. However, the use of testosterone in women is a subject of ongoing research and requires careful consideration.

- **Vaginal Rejuvenation Procedures:** Innovative procedures, such as laser therapy or radiofrequency treatments, aim to rejuvenate the vaginal tissues by stimulating collagen production and improving blood flow. These interventions can contribute to enhanced vaginal health and comfort.

- **Psychological Interventions:** Cognitive-behavioral therapy (CBT) or mindfulness-based interventions can address psychological factors influencing sexual health. These therapeutic approaches help individuals manage stress, anxiety, or negative thought patterns that may impact sexual well-being.

- **Regular Gynecological Check-ups:** Regular check-ups with a gynecologist are essential for monitoring pelvic health and discussing any concerns related to sexual function. Gynecologists can offer guidance, perform necessary screenings, and recommend appropriate interventions based on individual health profiles.

- **Medications for Sexual Desire:** Some medications designed to address hypoactive sexual desire disorder (HSDD) may be prescribed for post-menopausal women experiencing a persistent lack of sexual interest. These medications aim to enhance sexual desire and satisfaction.

CHAPTER FOURTEEN

AGING GRACEFULLY: BEAUTY AND SELF-CARE

Skin changes during menopause are a common and natural part of the aging process for women. The hormonal fluctuations, specifically the decline in estrogen levels, contribute to various changes in the skin's appearance, texture, and overall health. Understanding these changes and adopting appropriate skincare practices are essential for maintaining healthy and radiant skin during and after menopause.

1. **Loss of Elasticity and Collagen:** Estrogen plays a crucial role in maintaining the production of collagen and elastin, which provide the skin with its firmness and elasticity. During menopause, the decline in estrogen levels leads to a reduction in collagen production, resulting in skin laxity and the formation of wrinkles and fine lines.
2. **Thinning of the Skin:** The skin undergoes a thinning process during menopause due to decreased collagen and elastin. This thinning may

make the skin more susceptible to damage, bruising, and a translucent appearance.

3. **Dryness and Reduced Hydration:** Estrogen is also involved in maintaining the skin's natural moisture by influencing oil production. Reduced estrogen levels can lead to dryness and increased sensitivity. Dry skin is more prone to irritation, redness, and the development of rough patches.

4. **Increased Pigmentation:** Hormonal changes can stimulate melanin production, leading to increased pigmentation in certain areas of the skin. This may result in the development of age spots, dark patches (melasma), or uneven skin tone.

5. **Acne and Breakouts:** Some women may experience an onset or exacerbation of acne during menopause. Hormonal fluctuations can affect sebum production, leading to clogged pores and breakouts.

6. **Reduction in Skin Renewal and Healing:**

7. The skin's ability to renew and heal itself slows down with age. This, combined with hormonal changes, can result in a slower recovery from wounds, scars, and other skin imperfections.

8. **Increased Sensitivity:** Changes in hormone levels can make the skin more sensitive, prone to irritation, and reactive to skincare products. Women may find that they need to adjust their

skincare routine to accommodate these sensitivities.

Skincare Tips for Menopausal Skin:

Hydration:

Use moisturizers that are rich in hydrating ingredients like hyaluronic acid to combat dryness and maintain skin suppleness.

Sun Protection:

Prioritize sun protection by using a broad-spectrum sunscreen with an SPF of at least 30. Protecting the skin from harmful UV rays helps prevent premature aging and pigmentation.

Gentle Cleansing:

Opt for gentle, hydrating cleansers to avoid stripping the skin of its natural oils. Harsh cleansers can exacerbate dryness and sensitivity.

Anti-Aging Ingredients:

Include skincare products containing anti-aging ingredients such as retinoids, peptides, and antioxidants to stimulate collagen production and minimize the appearance of fine lines.

Exfoliation:

Incorporate gentle exfoliation into your routine to promote skin renewal. This can help with the removal of dead skin cells and improve the skin's texture.

Hydrating Masks:

Treat your skin to hydrating masks or treatments containing ingredients like aloe vera, chamomile, or glycerin to soothe and nourish.

Healthy Lifestyle Choices:

Maintain a healthy lifestyle by staying hydrated, eating a balanced diet rich in antioxidants, and getting regular exercise. These factors contribute to overall skin health.

Consultation with a Dermatologist:

If you experience persistent skin issues or concerns, consult with a dermatologist. They can provide personalized advice and recommend specific treatments or procedures tailored to your skin's needs.

Hormone Replacement Therapy (HRT):

For some women, hormone replacement therapy may be considered under the guidance of a healthcare professional. HRT can help address certain skin changes associated with hormonal fluctuations.

Hair And Nail Health

As women transition through the menopausal phase, the journey towards aging gracefully involves a holistic approach to beauty and self-care. Among the various aspects of well-being, maintaining healthy hair and nails is integral to fostering a sense of confidence and vitality during this transformative period. Let's delve into the nuances of nurturing hair and nail health as part of the broader theme of aging gracefully during menopause.

1. **Hormonal Influence on Hair and Nails:** Menopause heralds a decline in estrogen levels, impacting the health of both hair and nails. Understanding the hormonal nuances is crucial for tailoring care routines that address specific needs emerging during this phase.

2. **Hair Texture and Style Adaptation:** Changes in hormonal levels may manifest in shifts in hair texture. Embracing these changes might involve adapting hairstyles to suit the evolving needs of the hair, opting for styles that enhance volume or ease of management.

3. **Scalp and Hair Care Rituals:** Gentle care becomes paramount for maintaining a healthy scalp and hair. Moisturizing shampoos, regular conditioning,

and periodic treatments for hydration and nourishment contribute to overall hair vitality.

4. **Embracing Natural Beauty:** Aging gracefully involves embracing the natural beauty that comes with experience. Letting hair transition to its natural color, be it gray or silver, is a choice that aligns with the narrative of embracing one's unique journey.

5. **Nail Strength and Resilience:** Hormonal changes may impact the strength and resilience of nails. Implementing a nail care routine that includes gentle filing, moisturizing, and protection from harsh chemicals helps mitigate potential issues.

6. **Adequate Nutrition for Hair and Nails:** A well-balanced diet rich in proteins, vitamins, and minerals is fundamental for supporting the health of both hair and nails. Nutrients like biotin, iron, and omega-3 fatty acids contribute to their strength and luster.

7. **Regular Exercise for Circulation:** Engaging in regular physical activity not only promotes overall health but also supports good blood circulation, which is vital for delivering nutrients to hair follicles and nail beds, fostering their health.

8. **Hydration for Hair and Nails:** Maintaining adequate hydration is essential for the health of both hair and nails. Drinking enough water and

using hydrating products contribute to preventing dryness and promoting a vibrant appearance.

9. **Professional Guidance:** Seeking advice from professionals such as dermatologists or hairstylists specializing in mature hair care can provide personalized insights and recommendations tailored to individual needs.

10. **Mindful Stress Management:** Menopause can be a stressful phase, and stress can impact hair and nail health. Incorporating stress management techniques like meditation, mindfulness, or hobbies can contribute to overall well-being.

11. **Self-Care Rituals:** Establishing self-care rituals that involve pampering hair and nails can be both therapeutic and indulgent. This might include occasional deep conditioning treatments, manicures, or simply taking time for relaxation.

12. **Confidence in Self-Expression:** Embracing the changes in hair and nails with confidence fosters a positive self-image. Experimenting with different styles, colors, or nail art can be empowering, allowing women to express their unique personalities.

Positive Body Image In The Aging Process

As women navigate the transformative phase of menopause, embracing positive body image becomes a cornerstone of aging gracefully. Menopause, often accompanied by changes in hormonal levels and shifts in physical appearance, is an opportune time for women to redefine beauty, prioritize self-care, and foster a healthy relationship with their bodies. Here, we delve into the importance of cultivating a positive body image during the aging process, specifically focusing on menopause.

1. **Self-Acceptance and Appreciation:** Aging gracefully begins with cultivating self-acceptance and appreciation for the body's resilience through the years. Acknowledging the natural changes that come with menopause and viewing them as a testament to a life well-lived fosters a positive mindset.

2. **Redefined Notions of Beauty:** Menopause challenges conventional notions of beauty, emphasizing that true beauty is not confined to youthfulness. Embracing wrinkles, gray hair, and changes in body shape as symbols of wisdom and experience contributes to a more expansive and inclusive definition of beauty.

3. **Health-Centric Focus:** Shifting the focus from external appearance to overall health and well-being is paramount during menopause. Engaging in regular physical activity, adopting a nutritious diet, and prioritizing mental health are vital components of aging gracefully.

4. **Cultural and Media Literacy:** Understanding and challenging societal expectations perpetuated by media regarding beauty and aging is crucial. Actively seeking diverse representations of beauty in different ages and body types fosters a more inclusive perspective.

5. **Mind-Body Connection:** Nurturing the mind-body connection through practices like mindfulness, meditation, or yoga can enhance self-awareness and contribute to a positive perception of the body. These practices promote inner harmony and self-love.

6. **Fashion and Personal Style:** Redefining personal style and experimenting with fashion choices that reflect individuality can be empowering during menopause. Embracing one's unique style, irrespective of societal norms, contributes to a positive self-image.

7. **Self-Care Rituals:** Implementing self-care rituals tailored to individual preferences promotes a sense of well-being. This may include skincare routines, spa treatments, or activities that bring joy and

relaxation, contributing to a positive perception of the aging body.

8. **Community and Support:** Building a supportive community of friends and loved ones creates a space for shared experiences and mutual encouragement. Connecting with others who are navigating menopause reinforces positive body image through shared wisdom and understanding.

9. **Celebration of Achievements:** Menopause is a milestone, and celebrating the achievements and life experiences that have shaped a woman's journey fosters a sense of pride and confidence in her evolving identity.

10. **Educational Empowerment:** Knowledge about the physiological changes that occur during menopause empowers women to navigate this phase with resilience. Understanding that these changes are natural and universal reduces the impact of societal pressures on body image.

11. **Media Detox:** Taking breaks from media that perpetuate unrealistic beauty standards can be liberating. A media detox allows women to focus on their own journey, free from external judgments or comparisons.

12. **Gratitude Practice:** Incorporating a daily gratitude practice helps shift the focus towards positive aspects of life, fostering a sense of contentment and appreciation for the body and its capabilities.

CHAPTER FIFTEEN

INTEGRATIVE APPROACHES TO WOMEN'S HEALTH

Holistic Healthcare Models

In the realm of women's health, embracing an integrative approach involves considering the whole person—mind, body, and spirit—rather than solely focusing on symptoms or specific health concerns. Holistic healthcare models, as a key component of this integrative philosophy, emphasize the interconnectedness of various aspects of a woman's well-being. Here, we delve into the principles and benefits of holistic healthcare within the broader context of integrative approaches to women's health.

- **Definition of Holistic Healthcare:** Holistic healthcare is an inclusive approach that recognizes the intricate interplay of physical, mental, emotional, and spiritual dimensions of health. It views the individual as a complex, integrated system and seeks to address underlying causes rather than merely treating symptoms.
- **Person-Centered Care:** At the core of holistic healthcare is a person-centered approach. It values

the unique experiences, beliefs, and goals of each woman, recognizing that individualized care is essential for promoting overall well-being.

- **Mind-Body-Spirit Connection:** Holistic models acknowledge the interconnectedness of the mind, body, and spirit. Mental and emotional well-being are considered integral to physical health, and vice versa. Practices that promote balance and harmony across these dimensions are emphasized.

- **Preventive Care:** Holistic healthcare places a strong emphasis on preventive care. By addressing lifestyle factors, promoting healthy habits, and fostering resilience, the goal is to prevent illness and support women in maintaining optimal health throughout their lives.

- **Alternative Therapies and Complementary Medicine:** Integrating alternative therapies and complementary medicine is a hallmark of holistic healthcare. This may include practices such as acupuncture, herbal medicine, massage, yoga, and meditation, providing additional tools for managing health concerns.

- **Nutritional and Lifestyle Guidance:** Holistic healthcare models often incorporate personalized nutritional and lifestyle guidance. Recognizing the impact of diet, exercise, and stress management on overall health, women are empowered to make informed choices that support their well-being.

- **Mindfulness and Stress Reduction:** Mindfulness practices, including meditation and stress reduction techniques, are integral to holistic healthcare. These tools not only address mental and emotional aspects but also contribute to physical health by mitigating the effects of chronic stress.

- **Collaboration and Team-Based Care:** Holistic healthcare often involves collaboration among a team of healthcare professionals. This may include conventional medical practitioners, naturopaths, nutritionists, mental health professionals, and other specialists working together to address diverse aspects of a woman's health.

- **Emphasis on Education and Empowerment:** Holistic healthcare places a premium on education, empowering women with knowledge about their bodies, health conditions, and treatment options. This enables informed decision-making and active participation in their own care.

- **Cultural Competency:** Recognizing and respecting diverse cultural backgrounds and belief systems is intrinsic to holistic healthcare. Culturally competent care ensures that interventions align with individual values, promoting trust and collaboration between healthcare providers and women.

- **Holistic Approaches to Reproductive Health:** In the context of women's health, holistic models extend to reproductive health, recognizing the interconnected nature of hormonal, emotional, and physical factors. This includes approaches to fertility, pregnancy, and menopause that consider the broader well-being of women.
- **Continuous Evaluation and Adjustment:** Holistic healthcare is a dynamic process that involves continuous evaluation and adjustment of care plans. Recognizing that health is ever-evolving, holistic models allow for flexibility and responsiveness to changing needs.

Nutrition And Supplements

Integrative approaches to women's health encompass a holistic perspective that integrates conventional medicine with complementary therapies. Nutrition and supplements play a pivotal role in this paradigm, offering a foundation for overall well-being, addressing specific health concerns, and supporting women through various life stages. Here, we explore the detailed and comprehensive aspects of incorporating nutrition and supplements into integrative approaches for women's health.

- **Foundational Nutrition:** The cornerstone of integrative women's health is a balanced and nutrient-dense diet. Prioritizing a variety of whole foods, including fruits, vegetables, whole grains, lean proteins, and healthy fats, provides essential vitamins and minerals crucial for overall health.

- **Hormonal Balance through Diet:** Nutrition plays a significant role in maintaining hormonal balance, particularly during stages like menstruation, pregnancy, and menopause. Consuming foods rich in omega-3 fatty acids, phytoestrogens, and antioxidants can support hormonal health.

- **Bone Health and Calcium Intake:** Women, especially post-menopausal, are susceptible to bone-related issues. Adequate calcium intake, along with vitamin D and magnesium, is vital for maintaining bone density. Dairy products, leafy greens, and fortified foods are excellent dietary sources.

- **Iron and Anemia Prevention:** Iron-rich foods, such as lean meats, legumes, and leafy greens, are crucial to prevent iron deficiency anemia, a common concern for menstruating women. Combining iron-rich foods with vitamin C enhances absorption.

- **Folate and Pregnancy:** For women planning or in the early stages of pregnancy, sufficient folate intake is critical for fetal development. Leafy greens, fortified cereals, and legumes are excellent dietary sources.

- **Anti-Inflammatory Diet:** Chronic inflammation is associated with various women's health issues, including polycystic ovary syndrome (PCOS) and endometriosis. Adopting an anti-inflammatory diet, rich in fruits, vegetables, and omega-3 fatty acids, may provide relief.
- **Supplements for Specific Needs:** Targeted supplements can address specific health concerns. For example, omega-3 supplements may benefit heart health, while iron or vitamin B12 supplements can help correct deficiencies.
- **Probiotics for Gut Health:** The gut microbiome plays a crucial role in women's health, influencing digestion, immunity, and even mood. Probiotics, found in fermented foods or supplements, support a healthy gut microbiome.
- **Herbal Supplements:** Herbal supplements, like black cohosh for menopausal symptoms or chasteberry for menstrual irregularities, are components of integrative approaches. However, consultation with a healthcare professional is essential due to potential interactions.
- **Adaptogens for Stress Management:** Adaptogenic herbs, such as ashwagandha or Rhodiola, are believed to help the body adapt to stress.

Integrating adaptogens into the diet or as supplements may aid in stress management.

- **Collagen for Skin Health:** Collagen supplements are popular for supporting skin health and elasticity. While dietary sources include bone broth and fish, supplements are also available to enhance collagen intake.

- **Vitamin and Mineral Testing:** Periodic testing for vitamin and mineral levels ensures personalized supplementation. Testing helps identify deficiencies, guiding healthcare providers in recommending appropriate supplements.

- **Consultation with Healthcare Professionals:** Before incorporating supplements, women should consult with healthcare professionals. Individual health needs, potential interactions with medications, and personalized recommendations can be addressed through informed consultation.

Acupuncture And Alternative Therapies

Integrative approaches to women's health encompass a diverse range of modalities that extend beyond conventional medical practices. Among these, acupuncture and alternative therapies play a significant role in promoting holistic well-being. In the context of women's health, particularly addressing concerns related to menstruation, menopause, and reproductive health, acupuncture and alternative therapies offer unique perspectives and potential benefits. Here, we delve into the comprehensive understanding of how these practices contribute to the overall health and vitality of women.

1. Acupuncture:

Acupuncture, a traditional Chinese medicine practice, involves the insertion of thin needles into specific points on the body. In the context of women's health, acupuncture has shown promise in addressing various conditions:

- **Menstrual Irregularities:** Acupuncture may help regulate menstrual cycles and alleviate symptoms of premenstrual syndrome (PMS) by promoting hormonal balance.

- **Menopausal Symptoms:** Some women find relief from menopausal symptoms such as hot flashes, night sweats, and mood swings through acupuncture. It is believed to influence the balance of Yin and Yang energies in the body.

- **Fertility Support:** Acupuncture is often used as a complementary therapy for women undergoing fertility treatments. It may enhance blood flow to the reproductive organs and reduce stress, potentially improving fertility outcomes.

- **Pain Management:** Acupuncture is known for its analgesic effects and may be used to manage menstrual pain, pelvic pain, and other gynecological discomforts.

2. Herbal Medicine:

Herbal medicine, often used in conjunction with acupuncture, involves the use of plant-based remedies to address various health concerns. In women's health, herbal medicine is employed for:

- **Menstrual Health:** Certain herbs are believed to support menstrual regularity and alleviate symptoms associated with menstruation, such as cramps and bloating.
- **Menopausal Support:** Herbal remedies may be used to manage menopausal symptoms. For example, black cohosh is known for its potential to alleviate hot flashes.
- **Fertility Enhancement:** Herbal formulations may be prescribed to support reproductive health and address specific fertility concerns.

3. Meditation and Mindfulness:

Integrative approaches emphasize the connection between mental and physical health. Practices such as meditation and mindfulness play a crucial role in women's health by:

- **Stress Reduction:** Chronic stress can impact hormonal balance and contribute to menstrual

irregularities. Mindfulness practices help manage stress, promoting overall well-being.
- **Emotional Well-being during Menopause:** Meditation and mindfulness can assist women in navigating the emotional challenges associated with menopause, promoting a positive mindset.

4. Yoga and Movement Therapies:

Physical activity, including yoga and movement therapies, contributes to women's health in several ways:
- **Hormonal Balance:** Regular physical activity, such as yoga, is associated with hormonal balance, which can positively impact menstrual regularity.
- **Bone Health:** Weight-bearing exercises, including certain yoga poses, support bone health, addressing concerns related to osteoporosis in postmenopausal women.
- **Pelvic Health:** Yoga practices may enhance pelvic floor strength, promoting urinary and reproductive health.

5. Dietary and Nutritional Guidance:

Integrative approaches include personalized dietary and nutritional guidance:
- **Hormonal Support:** Certain foods and dietary patterns are believed to support hormonal balance,

addressing issues related to menstruation and menopause.

- **Fertility Nutrition:** Nutrition plays a crucial role in fertility. Integrative practitioners may offer guidance on dietary choices that support reproductive health.

6. Aromatherapy:

Aromatherapy involves the use of essential oils to promote well-being. In women's health, aromatherapy may be employed for:

- **Stress Reduction:** Certain scents, such as lavender or chamomile, are believed to have calming effects, aiding in stress reduction.
- **Sleep Support:** Aromatherapy can be used to create a relaxing environment, potentially improving sleep quality during various phases of a woman's life.

7. Chiropractic Care:

Chiropractic care focuses on the musculoskeletal system and its impact on overall health:

- **Pelvic Alignment:** Chiropractic adjustments may help address pelvic misalignments, offering relief from menstrual pain and supporting reproductive health.
- **Posture and Comfort:** Maintaining proper spinal alignment through chiropractic care contributes to

overall comfort, especially during pregnancy and postpartum.

8. Energy Healing Practices:

Practices such as Reiki or Qigong work with the body's energy fields:

- **Balance and Harmony:** Energy healing aims to restore balance and harmony in the body, potentially supporting overall well-being, including aspects of women's health.

9. Physical Therapy:

Physical therapy, when integrated into women's health practices, can address musculoskeletal issues and enhance overall well-being:

- **Pelvic Floor Rehabilitation:** Physical therapists specializing in pelvic health can provide exercises and techniques to improve pelvic floor function, addressing concerns such as incontinence and pelvic pain.
- **Prenatal and Postpartum Care:** Physical therapy supports women during pregnancy and postpartum, addressing musculoskeletal changes, promoting optimal positioning, and aiding in recovery.

10. Art and Expressive Therapies:

Creative and expressive therapies provide avenues for emotional expression and self-discovery:

- **Emotional Release:** Art and expressive therapies can serve as outlets for emotional expression, particularly useful for women navigating the emotional aspects of menopause.
- **Mind-Body Connection:** Engaging in creative activities fosters a connection between the mind and body, contributing to overall well-being.

11. Hydrotherapy:

Hydrotherapy involves the use of water for therapeutic purposes and can be beneficial in women's health:

- **Menstrual Pain Relief:** Warm baths or hydrotherapy techniques may offer relief from menstrual cramps and muscle tension.
- **Stress Reduction:** Immersion in water has relaxing effects, contributing to stress reduction and promoting a sense of calm.

12. Biofeedback:

Biofeedback involves using electronic monitoring to provide information about physiological processes, aiding in self-regulation:

- **Stress Management:** Biofeedback techniques can assist women in managing stress by providing

real-time feedback on physiological responses, promoting relaxation.
- **Pelvic Floor Health:** In the context of women's health, biofeedback may be used for pelvic floor rehabilitation, helping women gain awareness and control over these muscles.

13. Functional Medicine:

Functional medicine takes a holistic approach to address the root causes of health issues:
- **Hormonal Balancing:** Functional medicine practitioners may focus on addressing hormonal imbalances through personalized nutrition, lifestyle modifications, and targeted supplementation.
- **Gut Health:** Considering the gut-brain-hormone axis is crucial in functional medicine, as imbalances in gut health can impact hormonal regulation and overall well-being.

CHAPTER SIXTEEN

NAVIGATING MENOPAUSE IN THE WORKPLACE

Supporting Women In The Workforce

As awareness grows regarding the impact of menopause on women's health, there is an increasing need for organizations to create supportive environments that acknowledge and address the challenges women may face during this life stage. Navigating menopause in the workplace requires a comprehensive approach that fosters understanding, promotes inclusivity, and provides practical support. Here, we delve into strategies and considerations for supporting women in the workforce during the menopausal transition.

1. **Education and Awareness:** Creating awareness about menopause is crucial for fostering understanding among colleagues, supervisors, and HR personnel. Training programs and workshops can help dispel myths, reduce stigma, and encourage open conversations about menopause-related issues.

2. **Inclusive Policies:** Organizations should consider implementing inclusive policies that recognize the unique needs of menopausal women. This may include flexible work hours, remote work options, and adjustments to workplace temperature and lighting to accommodate the potential discomfort associated with menopausal symptoms.

3. **Open Communication Channels:** Establishing open communication channels allows women to discuss their experiences and needs without fear of judgment. Encouraging a culture where employees feel comfortable talking about menopause promotes a supportive and understanding work environment.

4. **Wellness Programs:** Integrating wellness programs that focus on holistic health can benefit menopausal women. Programs may include stress management workshops, nutrition seminars, and fitness classes designed to address the physical and emotional aspects of menopause.

5. **Employee Assistance Programs (EAPs):** EAPs can provide confidential support for employees experiencing challenges related to menopause. Offering counseling services and resources through EAPs can be valuable for women seeking assistance in managing the emotional and psychological aspects of this life stage.

6. **Flexible Working Arrangements:** Recognizing that menopausal symptoms can vary in intensity and duration, providing flexible working arrangements allows women to adapt their schedules to better manage their well-being. This flexibility may involve adjusted start and end times, compressed workweeks, or the option for part-time work.

7. **Menopause-Friendly Spaces:** Creating designated spaces within the workplace where women can take a break, rest, or engage in relaxation exercises can contribute to their overall well-being. These spaces should be comfortable, private, and equipped with amenities such as fans or cooling devices.

8. **Manager Training:** Training managers to recognize and understand menopausal symptoms enables them to provide appropriate support. This includes being aware of the potential impact on performance, offering flexibility when needed, and fostering a culture of empathy and understanding.

9. **Health Insurance Coverage:** Reviewing health insurance policies to ensure they cover treatments and therapies that may be beneficial for managing menopausal symptoms is essential. This may include coverage for hormone replacement therapy, counseling services, or alternative therapies.

10. **Supportive Peer Networks:** Encouraging the formation of peer support networks within the workplace allows women to share experiences, coping strategies, and tips for navigating menopause. Peer support fosters a sense of camaraderie and reduces feelings of isolation.
11. **Temperature Control:** Considering temperature control in the workplace, such as adjustable thermostats or localized cooling options, can help address the discomfort caused by hot flashes, a common symptom during menopause.
12. **Continued Professional Development:** Providing opportunities for continued professional development ensures that women going through menopause feel supported in their career growth. This can include mentorship programs, skill-building workshops, and networking events.
13. **Recognition and Acknowledgment:** Acknowledging the contributions of menopausal women to the workforce and recognizing their resilience during this transitional phase fosters a positive and appreciative workplace culture.

Accommodations And Policies

In the dynamic landscape of today's workforce, acknowledging and accommodating diverse needs is paramount to creating an inclusive and supportive environment. Accommodations and policies play a pivotal role in ensuring that employees, with varying requirements and life stages, can thrive in the workplace.

I.   Accommodations:

1. **Flexible Work Arrangements:** Offering flexible work arrangements, such as remote work options, flexible hours, or compressed workweeks, acknowledges the diverse needs of employees. This accommodation is particularly valuable for individuals managing caregiving responsibilities, health conditions, or navigating life stages such as parenthood or menopause.
2. **Accessible Workspaces:** Designing and maintaining accessible workspaces ensures that individuals with physical disabilities can navigate the workplace comfortably. This includes features such as ramps, elevators, ergonomic furniture, and considerations for individuals with sensory sensitivities.
3. **Technology Accommodations:** Providing technological accommodations, such as screen readers, speech-to-text software, or specialized keyboards, supports employees with disabilities

and ensures equitable access to information and communication tools.

4. **Training and Development Opportunities:** Accommodations in training and development programs recognize diverse learning styles and preferences. This may involve offering multiple learning formats, providing additional time for assessments, or creating inclusive materials that cater to various learning needs.

5. **Health and Wellness Programs:** Implementing health and wellness programs accommodates employees' holistic well-being. These programs may include fitness classes, mental health resources, stress management workshops, and initiatives that cater to the diverse health needs of the workforce.

6. **Lactation Rooms and Parental Support:** Recognizing the needs of working parents, especially new mothers, includes providing lactation rooms and parental support policies. These accommodations contribute to a family-friendly workplace and support the work-life balance of employees.

7. **Cultural Sensitivity and Inclusivity Training:** Accommodations in the form of cultural sensitivity and inclusivity training ensure that the workplace is respectful and inclusive of diverse backgrounds, fostering a sense of belonging among employees.

8. **Job Sharing and Part-Time Options:** Offering job-sharing arrangements and part-time work options accommodates individuals seeking more flexible work hours, allowing them to balance professional commitments with personal responsibilities or pursue other interests.

II. Policies:

1. **Diversity and Inclusion Policy:** A well-defined diversity and inclusion policy communicates the organization's commitment to creating a diverse and inclusive workplace. This policy should encompass hiring practices, promotion opportunities, and a zero-tolerance approach to discrimination.
2. **Equal Opportunity Employment Policy:** An equal opportunity employment policy ensures that all employees, regardless of their background, have an equal chance for career advancement and are not subjected to discrimination based on gender, race, age, disability, or other protected characteristics.
3. **Anti-Harassment and Anti-Discrimination Policies:** Establishing clear anti-harassment and anti-discrimination policies is essential for maintaining a respectful and safe workplace. These policies should outline reporting procedures and

consequences for violations, creating a culture of accountability.

4. **Remote Work Policy:** A well-structured remote work policy provides guidelines for employees working outside the traditional office setting. It addresses expectations, communication protocols, and outlines the eligibility criteria and approval process for remote work arrangements.

5. **Family and Medical Leave Policy:** A comprehensive family and medical leave policy ensures that employees can take necessary leave for family-related or medical reasons without fear of repercussions. This policy often includes provisions for maternity and paternity leave, caregiving responsibilities, and medical emergencies.

6. **Accommodation Request Procedures:** Clearly defining procedures for accommodation requests ensures a transparent and accessible process for employees seeking accommodations. This includes outlining how requests should be made, the information required, and the organization's commitment to confidentiality.

7. **Workplace Flexibility Policy:** A workplace flexibility policy sets the foundation for accommodating diverse work arrangements. It outlines the organization's approach to flexibility, including expectations, communication protocols,

and the benefits associated with flexible work options.

8. **Education and Training Policies:** Policies related to education and training ensure that employees have access to continuous learning opportunities. These policies may include guidelines for professional development, reimbursement for educational expenses, and expectations for ongoing skill enhancement.

9. **Privacy and Confidentiality Policy:** A privacy and confidentiality policy safeguards employees' personal information and ensures that sensitive details related to accommodation requests, health issues, or personal circumstances are handled with the utmost discretion and compliance with privacy laws.

10. **Return-to-Work Policies:** Establishing clear return-to-work policies supports employees transitioning back to work after a leave of absence, whether for medical reasons, parental leave, or other personal circumstances. These policies provide a structured framework for reintegration and may include phased returns or flexible schedules.

Mental Health And Work-Life Balance

In the fast-paced and demanding landscape of the modern workplace, maintaining mental health and achieving a sustainable work-life balance are paramount for overall well-being and professional success. As our understanding of mental health deepens, employers and employees alike are recognizing the profound impact that work-life balance has on mental well-being.

Understanding Mental Health in the Workplace: Mental health encompasses emotional, psychological, and social well-being, influencing how individuals think, feel, and act. In the workplace, factors such as job satisfaction, workload, interpersonal relationships, and organizational culture significantly impact mental health. A supportive work environment recognizes the importance of mental well-being and actively promotes practices that enhance it.

The Impact of Work on Mental Health: Work-related stress, pressure, and long working hours can contribute to mental health challenges. It is essential to recognize the signs of mental health issues, including burnout, anxiety, and depression, and address them proactively to create a healthier workplace culture.

Promoting Mental Health at Work: Employers can take proactive steps to promote mental health in the workplace:

- **Mental Health Programs:** Implementing mental health programs that raise awareness, provide resources, and destigmatize seeking help can create a supportive environment.
- **Training and Education:** Offering training sessions on stress management, resilience building, and mental health first aid equips employees with tools to navigate challenges effectively.
- **Access to Counseling Services:** Providing access to confidential counseling services allows employees to seek professional support when facing mental health concerns.

Work-Life Balance Defined: Work-life balance is the equilibrium between professional responsibilities and personal life. Achieving balance fosters a sense of fulfillment, reduces stress, and enhances overall well-being. Striking the right balance contributes to increased productivity, job satisfaction, and employee retention.

Challenges to Work-Life Balance: Various factors can disrupt work-life balance:

- **Excessive Workload:** Unrealistic workloads and tight deadlines can lead to long working hours, impacting personal time and well-being.
- **Lack of Flexibility:** Inflexible work schedules may hinder employees from managing personal commitments or achieving a harmonious work-life balance.
- **Technological Intrusion:** Constant connectivity through technology can blur the boundaries between work and personal life, making it challenging for individuals to disconnect.

Strategies for Fostering Work-Life Balance: Employers and employees can collaborate to create a work environment that prioritizes work-life balance:

- **Flexible Work Arrangements:** Offering flexible work hours, remote work options, or compressed workweeks allows employees to tailor their schedules to better align with personal commitments.
- **Clear Communication:** Establishing clear communication channels regarding expectations, deadlines, and boundaries helps manage work-related stress and promotes a healthy work culture.
- **Encouraging Breaks:** Encouraging regular breaks, including lunch breaks and short walks, supports mental well-being and contributes to increased productivity.

- **Time Management Training:** Providing training on effective time management empowers employees to prioritize tasks, set realistic goals, and avoid burnout.

The Role of Leadership: Leadership plays a crucial role in shaping the work environment and influencing the well-being of employees:

- **Leading by Example:** Leaders who prioritize their own work-life balance set a positive example for their teams, fostering a culture where balance is valued.
- **Supportive Leadership:** Leaders who are attuned to the needs of their team members and offer support during challenging times contribute to a positive and inclusive workplace.

Employee Well-Being Initiatives: Implementing employee well-being initiatives demonstrates a commitment to fostering a healthy work-life balance:\

- **Wellness Programs:** Offering wellness programs that address physical, mental, and emotional well-being, such as fitness classes, mindfulness sessions, and health workshops, contributes to a holistic approach.
- **Employee Assistance Programs (EAPs):** Providing access to EAPs for confidential counseling and

support services demonstrates a commitment to employees' mental health.

Personal Strategies for Employees: Employees also play an active role in managing their work-life balance:
- **Setting Boundaries:** Establishing clear boundaries between work and personal life, including designated workspaces and specific work hours, helps create a sense of separation.
- **Prioritizing Self-Care:** Prioritizing self-care activities, such as exercise, relaxation, and hobbies, contributes to overall well-being and resilience.
- **Effective Time Management:** Developing effective time management skills allows individuals to optimize their work hours and allocate time for personal pursuits.

The Business Case for Work-Life Balance: Fostering work-life balance is not only a matter of employee well-being but also makes good business sense:
- **Increased Productivity:** Employees with a balanced work-life schedule are more likely to be productive, focused, and engaged in their work.
- **Talent Attraction and Retention:** Organizations that prioritize work-life balance are more attractive to potential employees and are better positioned to retain top talent.

- **Reduced Absenteeism and Turnover:** A supportive work-life balance culture contributes to lower rates of absenteeism and turnover, saving on recruitment and training costs.

Remote Work and Work-Life Integration: The rise of remote work has reshaped traditional notions of work-life balance:

- **Flexible Location:** Remote work offers the flexibility to choose work locations, allowing employees to create environments that support their well-being.
- **Challenges of Boundaries:** Remote work, while providing flexibility, can also blur the lines between professional and personal life. Establishing clear boundaries is crucial.

Addressing Stigma and Culture Shift: Overcoming the stigma associated with taking breaks, working flexible hours, or seeking support for mental health challenges requires a cultural shift within organizations:

- **Promoting Inclusivity:** Fostering an inclusive culture where diverse needs are acknowledged and accommodated helps break down stigmas and encourages open conversations.
- **Leadership Advocacy:** Leaders advocating for work-life balance and mental health initiatives

signal to employees that these priorities are integral to the organizational culture.

Continuous Evaluation and Adaptation: Work-life balance is dynamic and subject to change based on individual needs, life stages, and external factors. Continuous evaluation and adaptation of policies and initiatives ensure they remain relevant and effective.

CHAPTER SEVENTEEN

FUTURE TRENDS IN MENOPAUSAL RESEARCH

Advancements In Hormonal Therapies

As the field of menopausal research evolves, groundbreaking advancements in hormonal therapies are paving the way for innovative approaches to managing menopausal symptoms and promoting women's health during this significant life stage. These advancements represent a dynamic shift in how menopause is understood and treated, ushering in a new era of personalized and targeted hormonal interventions. 3

1. **Precision Hormone Therapies:** Emerging research is steering towards precision medicine, tailoring hormonal therapies to individual needs. This approach involves assessing a woman's unique hormonal profile, genetic factors, and specific symptomatology to design a personalized hormone therapy regimen. Precision hormone therapies aim to optimize efficacy while minimizing potential risks, offering a more

nuanced and individualized approach to managing menopausal symptoms.

2. **Bioidentical Hormones:** Bioidentical hormones, derived from plant sources and designed to mimic the molecular structure of hormones produced in the human body, represent a growing area of interest in menopausal research. These hormones, including bioidentical estrogen and progesterone, aim to provide a more natural and physiologically aligned alternative to traditional hormone replacement therapies (HRT). Ongoing studies are investigating the safety and efficacy of bioidentical hormones in managing menopausal symptoms.

3. **Hormone Replacement Therapy Innovations:** Traditional hormone replacement therapy is undergoing innovative transformations to enhance safety and effectiveness. Research is focusing on developing novel delivery methods, such as transdermal patches, gels, and subcutaneous implants, aiming to achieve more stable hormone levels and reduce the risks associated with oral administration. Additionally, efforts are directed towards optimizing the combination and dosages of hormones in HRT for improved symptom control.

4. **Hormone Modulation Beyond Estrogen and Progesterone:** Beyond estrogen and progesterone, researchers are exploring the modulation of other

hormones to address a broader spectrum of menopausal symptoms. Investigational therapies targeting hormones such as dehydroepiandrosterone (DHEA), testosterone, and neuroactive steroids are being studied for their potential in alleviating symptoms such as sexual dysfunction, mood disturbances, and cognitive changes.

5. **Non-Hormonal Therapies:** Advancements in menopausal research extend beyond hormonal interventions to encompass non-hormonal therapies. Research is investigating the efficacy of selective serotonin and norepinephrine reuptake inhibitors (SSRIs and SNRIs), gabapentinoids, and other non-hormonal medications in managing vasomotor symptoms, sleep disturbances, and mood-related issues during menopause. These non-hormonal options provide alternatives for women who may not be suitable candidates for hormonal therapies.

6. **Nutraceuticals and Herbal Therapies:** The exploration of nutraceuticals and herbal therapies as adjuncts to conventional treatments is gaining momentum. Substances such as phytoestrogens, black cohosh, and red clover are being studied for their potential in managing menopausal symptoms. Additionally, research is delving into the role of

dietary supplements and lifestyle modifications in promoting overall well-being during menopause.

7. **Targeting Specific Symptom Clusters:** Advancements in research are directing attention towards understanding and targeting specific symptom clusters experienced by menopausal women. Tailoring interventions to address combinations of symptoms, such as vasomotor symptoms coupled with sleep disturbances or mood changes, allows for a more comprehensive and effective approach to menopausal care.

8. **Genomic and Proteomic Approaches:** Genomic and proteomic research is unraveling the intricate interplay of genetic and protein-level factors in menopause. Studying the genetic variations associated with hormone metabolism, receptor sensitivity, and symptom susceptibility allows for a deeper understanding of individualized responses to hormonal therapies. This knowledge contributes to the development of targeted interventions based on an individual's genetic and proteomic profile.

9. **Hormonal Therapies and Cardiovascular Health:** As cardiovascular health becomes a focal point in menopausal research, hormonal therapies are being scrutinized for their impact on heart health. Future trends involve refining hormonal interventions to minimize cardiovascular risks and

exploring novel therapies that may have positive effects on lipid profiles, vascular function, and overall cardiovascular well-being during and after menopause.

10. **Telehealth and Digital Interventions:** The integration of telehealth and digital interventions is revolutionizing menopausal care accessibility. From virtual consultations for personalized hormone therapy prescriptions to mobile applications providing symptom tracking and self-management tools, technology is enhancing the delivery of menopausal healthcare. These innovations empower women to actively engage in their well-being and access support remotely.

11. **Long-Term Safety and Efficacy Studies:** The commitment to ensuring the long-term safety and efficacy of hormonal therapies remains a cornerstone of menopausal research. Ongoing and future studies focus on extended follow-up periods to assess the sustained benefits and potential risks associated with various hormonal interventions, providing comprehensive data to guide clinical decision-making.

12. **Collaborative and Multidisciplinary Research:** Future trends in menopausal research emphasize collaborative and multidisciplinary approaches. Engaging researchers, clinicians, pharmacologists, and experts from diverse fields facilitates a holistic

understanding of menopause and encourages the development of integrated and comprehensive care models.

Innovative Approaches To Symptom Management

As the field of menopausal research evolves, exploring innovative approaches to symptom management has become a focal point in enhancing the quality of life for women navigating the menopausal transition. Future trends in menopausal research are marked by a commitment to advancing scientific understanding and developing novel interventions to address the diverse and often challenging symptoms associated with menopause. This comprehensive note delves into cutting-edge strategies and emerging trends in menopausal symptom management.

1. **Precision Medicine in Menopausal Symptom Management:** Harnessing the principles of precision medicine involves tailoring interventions based on individual characteristics such as genetics, hormonal profiles, and lifestyle factors. This approach aims to create personalized strategies for

symptom management that consider the unique biological makeup of each woman.

2. **Hormone Replacement Therapies (HRT) Reimagined:** The exploration of more refined and targeted hormone replacement therapies is a key area of future research. This includes developing customized hormone formulations, exploring alternative delivery methods, and optimizing dosages to maximize efficacy while minimizing potential risks.

3. **Neurocognitive Interventions:** Addressing cognitive symptoms associated with menopause, such as memory loss and cognitive decline, involves innovative neurocognitive interventions. Cognitive training programs, brain stimulation techniques, and pharmaceutical interventions are being explored to enhance cognitive function during and after menopause.

4. **Nutraceuticals and Functional Foods:** Investigating the role of nutraceuticals and functional foods in menopausal symptom management is gaining prominence. Research focuses on identifying specific dietary components and supplements that can alleviate symptoms, with an emphasis on their impact on hormonal balance, bone health, and cardiovascular function.

5. **Non-Hormonal Pharmacological Approaches:** The development of non-hormonal pharmacological

options for symptom management is a notable trend. This includes medications targeting specific neurotransmitter systems, inflammatory pathways, and other biological mechanisms to address symptoms like hot flashes, mood disturbances, and sleep disturbances.

6. **Integrative and Complementary Therapies:** Integrative approaches that combine conventional medicine with complementary therapies are gaining recognition. Techniques such as acupuncture, mindfulness-based stress reduction, and herbal supplements are being explored for their potential in managing menopausal symptoms and improving overall well-being.

7. **Wearable Technology for Symptom Monitoring:** Leveraging wearable technology for real-time symptom monitoring is a futuristic trend. Devices equipped with sensors can track physiological parameters, providing valuable data for understanding symptom patterns and tailoring interventions to individual needs.

8. **Telehealth and Digital Health Solutions:** The integration of telehealth and digital health solutions facilitates remote access to healthcare resources. Virtual consultations, mobile applications, and online platforms provide women with convenient access to information, support,

and personalized interventions for managing menopausal symptoms.

9. **Psychobehavioral Interventions:** Recognizing the intricate connection between psychological well-being and menopausal symptoms, psychobehavioral interventions are being explored. Cognitive-behavioral therapy, mindfulness-based approaches, and stress management techniques aim to alleviate mood disturbances and improve overall mental health.

10. **Genomic and Epigenetic Research:** Advancements in genomic and epigenetic research are shedding light on the genetic factors influencing menopausal symptoms. Understanding the interplay between genetics and environmental factors opens avenues for targeted interventions and precision medicine approaches.

11. **Microbiome Interventions:**Exploring the role of the gut microbiome in menopausal health is an emerging area of interest. Probiotics, prebiotics, and dietary interventions aimed at promoting a healthy gut microbiome are being investigated for their potential impact on menopausal symptoms.

12. **Mind-Body Therapies:** Integrating mind-body therapies such as yoga, tai chi, and biofeedback into menopausal symptom management is gaining traction. These approaches focus on the interconnectedness of physical and mental well-

being, offering holistic strategies for symptom relief.

13. **Environmental and Lifestyle Modifications:** Recognizing the influence of environmental factors on menopausal symptoms, future research includes exploring lifestyle modifications. This encompasses changes in diet, physical activity, sleep hygiene, and exposure to environmental toxins to optimize overall health during and after menopause.

Personalized Medicine In Menopausal Care

As the field of menopausal research advances, the concept of personalized medicine emerges as a promising avenue for tailoring menopausal care to individual needs, characteristics, and health profiles. Personalized medicine, also known as precision medicine, involves customizing medical interventions based on a person's unique genetic, biological, and lifestyle factors. In the context of menopausal care, this innovative approach holds the potential to revolutionize how healthcare providers address the diverse experiences and challenges women encounter during the menopausal transition.

1.   Understanding Menopausal Diversity:
Menopause is a complex and individualized experience influenced by a myriad of factors, including genetics, hormone levels, lifestyle, and overall health. Traditional approaches to menopausal care often adopt a one-size-fits-all model, overlooking the diversity in symptoms, treatment responses, and long-term health outcomes among women. Personalized medicine seeks to rectify this by acknowledging and addressing the unique aspects of each woman's menopausal journey.

2.   Genetic and Genomic Insights:
The integration of genetic and genomic information into menopausal care represents a key aspect of personalized medicine:

- **Genetic Variability:** Variations in specific genes can influence how women experience menopause and their susceptibility to certain symptoms or conditions.

- **Hormone Receptor Genes:** Genetic factors may impact how women respond to hormone replacement therapy (HRT), guiding healthcare providers in tailoring hormone interventions based on individual genetic profiles.

3.   Hormone Profiling:

Personalized medicine allows for comprehensive hormone profiling to understand the unique hormonal milieu of each woman:

- **Individual Hormone Levels:** Assessing individual hormone levels, including estrogen, progesterone, and testosterone, enables a more precise understanding of hormonal fluctuations during menopause.
- **Dynamic Monitoring:** Continuous monitoring of hormone levels facilitates real-time adjustments to hormone-based interventions, optimizing efficacy and minimizing side effects.

4. Lifestyle and Environmental Factors:

Personalized medicine in menopausal care extends beyond genetics to consider lifestyle and environmental factors:

- **Diet and Nutrition:** Tailoring dietary recommendations based on individual nutritional needs and preferences supports overall health and addresses specific menopausal concerns.
- **Physical Activity:** Personalized exercise plans can be designed to address bone health, cardiovascular fitness, and weight management, considering individual fitness levels and preferences.

5. Symptom-Based Approaches:

Instead of a generalized approach to managing menopausal symptoms, personalized medicine allows for targeted interventions based on specific symptoms:

- **Hot Flashes:** Tailored interventions, including hormone therapies or non-hormonal alternatives, can be recommended based on the severity and frequency of hot flashes.

- **Mood Disturbances:** Understanding an individual's mental health history and genetic predispositions allows for personalized strategies to address mood disturbances, such as anxiety or depression.

6. Individualized Risk Assessments:

Personalized medicine enables healthcare providers to conduct individualized risk assessments:

- **Cardiovascular Risk:** Considering factors such as blood pressure, cholesterol levels, and individual cardiovascular risk profiles allows for personalized cardiovascular health strategies.

- **Bone Health:** Personalized assessments of bone density and fracture risk guide interventions to support bone health, considering individual susceptibility to osteoporosis.

7. Integrative Approaches:

Personalized menopausal care emphasizes integrative approaches that consider the whole woman:

- **Complementary Therapies:** Integrating personalized recommendations for complementary therapies, such as acupuncture, herbal supplements, or mindfulness practices, aligns with individual preferences and needs.
- **Mind-Body Connection:** Recognizing the impact of stress and mental health on menopausal experiences allows for personalized strategies that prioritize emotional well-being.

8. **Advanced Diagnostic Technologies:**
The future of personalized menopausal care incorporates cutting-edge diagnostic technologies:

- **Biomarker Identification:** Identifying specific biomarkers associated with menopausal symptoms or health risks allows for early intervention and targeted treatments.
- **Non-Invasive Monitoring:** Advancements in non-invasive monitoring, such as wearable devices, provide real-time data on physiological parameters, aiding in personalized care plans.

9. **Patient Empowerment and Informed Decision-Making:** Personalized medicine empowers women to actively participate in their healthcare decisions:

- **Informed Choices:** Providing women with personalized information about their health, treatment options, and potential outcomes facilitates informed decision-making.

- **Shared Decision-Making:** Collaborative discussions between healthcare providers and women ensure that interventions align with individual preferences, values, and goals.

10. Ethical Considerations and Privacy:

The adoption of personalized medicine raises important ethical considerations:

- **Informed Consent:** Ensuring women are well-informed about the implications of genetic testing, hormone profiling, and other personalized approaches is crucial for obtaining informed consent.
- **Data Security:** Safeguarding the privacy and security of genetic and health data is paramount, necessitating robust measures to protect sensitive information.

11. Collaborative Research Initiatives:

The future of personalized menopausal care relies on collaborative research efforts:

- **Large-Scale Studies:** Conducting large-scale studies that incorporate diverse populations help identify commonalities and differences in menopausal experiences, contributing to more effective personalized interventions.

- **Multidisciplinary Research:** Integrating expertise from various fields, including genetics, endocrinology, psychology, and nutrition, fosters a holistic understanding of menopausal health.

12.   Digital Health Solutions:

Personalized menopausal care is likely to benefit from the widespread use of digital health solutions:

- **Mobile Apps:** Mobile applications that track symptoms, provide personalized recommendations, and facilitate communication between women and healthcare providers enhance the accessibility of personalized care.
- **Telemedicine:** Telemedicine platforms enable remote consultations, making personalized menopausal care more accessible to women in diverse geographic locations.

13. Implementation Challenges and Future Directions:

While personalized menopausal care holds great promise, challenges such as cost, accessibility, and integration into healthcare systems must be addressed. Future research should focus on overcoming these challenges and refining personalized approaches to maximize their impact on women's health and well-being.

CHAPTER EIGHTEEN

RESOURCES FOR WOMEN'S HEALTH

Support Groups And Communities

Navigating the intricate landscape of women's health is an individual journey often marked by unique challenges and experiences. Support groups and communities tailored to specific health concerns and life stages play an indispensable role in providing women with the tools, resources, and shared connections needed to traverse their health journeys. Let's look into a detailed exploration of diverse and comprehensive support groups and communities dedicated to enhancing women's health across various domains.

1.   Women's Health Foundation:
Focus: Encompasses a broad spectrum of women's health issues.
Platform: Offers both online community forums and in-person support groups.
Emphasis: Strives for holistic well-being through education, mutual support, and advocacy efforts.

2.   Breast Cancer Support Network:
Focus: Tailored for breast cancer survivors and those undergoing treatment.
Platform: Provides online forums, local chapter meetings, and virtual support groups.
Emphasis: Centers around emotional support, survivorship celebrations, and raising awareness.

3.   Postpartum Wellness Group:
Focus: Specifically addresses postpartum mental health and wellness.
Platform: Engages participants through a combination of in-person and online meetings.
Emphasis: Advocates for mental health, shares experiences, and explores coping strategies.

4.   Endometriosis Warriors Collective:
Focus: A supportive community for women grappling with endometriosis.
Platform: Establishes a presence through online forums, local meet-ups, and awareness events.
Emphasis: Advocates for awareness, educates on the condition, and fosters mutual support.

5.   Menopause Matters Community:
Focus: Tailored for menopausal women seeking support and information.

Platform: Utilizes online forums, webinars, and virtual support groups.
Emphasis: Addresses symptom management, lifestyle adjustments, and hormonal health during menopause.

6.   Autoimmune Sisters:

Focus: Designed for women managing various autoimmune disorders.
Platform: Offers an online community, local chapter meet-ups, and virtual events.
Emphasis: Promotes mutual support, shares lifestyle management tips, and advocates for autoimmune health.

7.   Depression and Anxiety Support Alliance for Women:

Focus: A community for women dealing with depression and anxiety.
Platform: Engages participants through online meetings, educational resources, and peer support.
Emphasis: Advocates for mental health awareness, shares coping strategies, and works toward reducing stigma.

8.   Fertility Friends Network:

Focus: Tailored for women navigating fertility challenges.

Platform: Utilizes online forums, virtual support groups, and informational webinars.
Emphasis: Offers emotional support, shared experiences, and educational resources on fertility.

9. Chronic Pain Warriors Circle:
Focus: Supports women managing chronic pain conditions.
Platform: Engages participants through virtual meetings, online resources, and community events.
Emphasis: Shares pain management strategies, offers emotional support, and provides lifestyle tips.

10. Gynecological Cancer Survivors Alliance:
Focus: A community for women survivors of gynecological cancers.
Platform: Utilizes in-person support groups, online forums, and awareness campaigns.
Emphasis: Celebrates survivorship, advocates for ongoing health, and provides support for post-cancer life.

11. Wellness Over 50:
Focus: Tailored for women over 50 navigating aging and health changes.
Platform: Establishes an online community, hosts virtual meet-ups, and offers wellness workshops.

Emphasis: Guides women in aging gracefully, provides health tips, and fosters peer support.

## 12.	Heart Health Women's Network:

Focus: Centers around cardiovascular health for women.

Platform: Engages participants through online forums, educational webinars, and local awareness events.

Emphasis: Encourages heart-healthy lifestyles, emphasizes prevention, and offers peer-to-peer encouragement.

## 13.	Women's Mental Health Collective:

Focus: Addresses mental health and wellness for women.

Platform: Utilizes online support groups, mindfulness sessions, and educational resources.

Emphasis: Prioritizes emotional well-being, works towards reducing stigma, and shares coping strategies.

Educational Materials And Websites

## 1.	Mayo Clinic Women's Health:

Website: Mayo Clinic Women's Health

Mayo Clinic, a renowned medical institution, offers an extensive online resource dedicated to women's health. The Mayo Clinic Women's Health website provides comprehensive information on various aspects of women's well-being. It covers topics such as reproductive health, nutrition, fitness, mental health, and preventive care. The content is evidence-based, created by medical professionals, and is easily accessible for women seeking reliable information to make informed decisions about their health. The website also features interactive tools, expert advice, and the latest research updates, making it a valuable resource for women of all ages.

2. Women's Health.gov:

Website: Women's Health.gov

Women's Health.gov, managed by the U.S. Department of Health and Human Services, is a comprehensive online platform offering evidence-based information on a wide range of women's health topics. The website covers areas such as reproductive health, pregnancy, mental health, and chronic conditions. It provides resources in English and Spanish, ensuring inclusivity. Women can find educational materials, fact sheets, and tools to support their health and well-being. The content is regularly updated to reflect the latest medical guidelines, making it a reliable source for women seeking trustworthy information.

3.   WebMD Women's Health:
Website: WebMD Women's Health

WebMD is a well-known health information platform, and its Women's Health section is dedicated to addressing the specific health concerns of women. The website offers a wealth of articles, expert advice, and interactive tools covering topics from reproductive health to mental well-being. WebMD's strength lies in its user-friendly interface, making complex medical information accessible to a broad audience. The content is regularly reviewed by healthcare professionals, ensuring accuracy and relevance for women seeking reliable health information.

4.   National Women's Health Network:
Website: National Women's Health Network

The National Women's Health Network is a non-profit organization focused on promoting women's health advocacy and providing evidence-based information. Their website serves as a hub for educational materials on various health issues affecting women. From reproductive rights to healthcare policy, the NWHN addresses critical topics to empower women to make informed decisions about their health. The organization also engages in advocacy work, making it a valuable resource for those interested in staying informed about women's health on a broader societal level.

5.   The American College of Obstetricians and Gynecologists (ACOG):
Website: ACOG Women's Health

ACOG, a leading professional association for obstetricians and gynecologists, provides a wealth of educational resources on its website. Aimed at both healthcare professionals and the general public, ACOG's Women's Health section covers topics ranging from prenatal care to menopause. The organization's commitment to evidence-based practice ensures that the information provided is reliable and up-to-date. Women can find patient education materials, guidelines, and news on emerging trends in women's healthcare.

6.   Centers for Disease Control and Prevention (CDC) - Women's Health:
Website: CDC Women's Health

The Centers for Disease Control and Prevention (CDC) dedicates a section of its website specifically to women's health, providing a wealth of resources and information. Covering a wide array of topics, including maternal health, chronic diseases, and preventive care, the CDC's Women's Health section is a go-to source for evidence-based content. The website features educational materials, statistical data, and guidelines, making it a reliable reference for women, healthcare professionals, and researchers alike.

7.   Women's Health Magazine:
Website: Women's Health Magazine

Women's Health Magazine is a popular publication that combines expert advice with accessible content on various aspects of women's well-being. The website features articles, fitness routines, nutrition tips, and mental health insights tailored to a diverse audience. Women can find information on lifestyle, beauty, and fitness, presented in an engaging and relatable format. While not a substitute for medical advice, Women's Health Magazine serves as a supplement to traditional health resources, offering practical tips for maintaining a healthy lifestyle.

8.   Mayo Clinic - Healthy Lifestyle: Women's Health:
Website: Mayo Clinic - Women's Health

Mayo Clinic's broader Healthy Lifestyle section includes a dedicated focus on women's health, providing evidence-based guidance on nutrition, fitness, mental well-being, and preventive care. The content is presented in a user-friendly format, making it accessible to a wide audience. Mayo Clinic's reputation for medical excellence ensures that the information is trustworthy and aligns with the latest medical research. Women can find practical advice and resources to support their health and well-being.

9.   Harvard Health - Women's Health Watch:
Website: Harvard Women's Health Watch

Harvard Health's Women's Health Watch is a publication that distills the expertise of Harvard Medical School into accessible and informative content. The website covers a spectrum of women's health topics, from reproductive health to aging. Articles are authored by medical professionals and researchers, ensuring a high standard of accuracy and reliability. Women seeking in-depth insights and evidence-based information will find Harvard Women's Health Watch to be a valuable resource.

10.   Office on Women's Health - U.S. Department of Health & Human Services:
Website: OWH - HHS

The Office on Women's Health, a branch of the U.S. Department of Health & Human Services, operates a comprehensive website dedicated to women's health. This resource covers a broad spectrum of topics, including reproductive health, mental health, and preventive care. The website provides educational materials, fact sheets, and tools to empower women to make informed decisions about their health. The content is regularly updated and reviewed by healthcare professionals, ensuring accuracy and relevance.

11. Johns Hopkins Medicine - Women's Health: **Website:** Johns Hopkins Women's Health

Johns Hopkins Medicine, a leading healthcare institution, provides a dedicated section on women's health on its website. This resource covers a wide range of topics, including gynecological health, reproductive medicine, and general well-being. The content is backed by the expertise of healthcare professionals at Johns Hopkins, ensuring reliability and accuracy. The website serves as a valuable reference for women seeking trustworthy information on various health aspects, from routine care to specialized medical concerns.

12. HealthyWomen:

Website: HealthyWomen

HealthyWomen is a non-profit organization committed to providing women with trustworthy health information. The website covers a diverse array of topics, including reproductive health, mental health, and lifestyle. With a focus on empowering women through education, HealthyWomen offers articles, webinars, and expert insights to support informed decision-making. The organization collaborates with healthcare professionals to ensure that the content aligns with current medical knowledge, making it a valuable resource for women seeking reliable health information.

13. Cleveland Clinic - Women's Health:
Website: Cleveland Clinic - Women's Health

The Cleveland Clinic, known for its medical expertise, provides a dedicated online resource focusing on women's health. Covering a wide range of topics, from gynecological care to heart health, the website offers evidence-based information in an easily accessible format. Women can find articles, videos, and tools designed to educate and empower. With a commitment to patient-centered care, the Cleveland Clinic's Women's Health section stands as a reliable source for women seeking information on maintaining and enhancing their well-being.

14.   Women's Heart Foundation:
Website: Women's Heart Foundation

The Women's Heart Foundation is dedicated to promoting women's heart health, addressing the unique aspects of cardiovascular health in women. The organization's website provides educational resources, information on heart disease prevention, and insights into women's cardiovascular research. With a focus on advocacy and awareness, the Women's Heart Foundation serves as a valuable resource for women looking to understand and prioritize their heart health.

15.   Planned Parenthood - Sexual & Reproductive Health:
Website: Planned Parenthood

Planned Parenthood is a prominent organization providing reproductive health services, including education and information on sexual health. Their website covers a wide range of topics, from contraception to sexually transmitted infections (STIs). Planned Parenthood offers comprehensive and inclusive resources for women of all ages, aiming to empower individuals to make informed choices about their sexual and reproductive health.

Healthcare Providers And Specialists

I. **Gynecologist:** Gynecologists specialize in the health of the female reproductive system. They provide preventive care, conduct screenings, manage reproductive health issues, and offer family planning services. Gynecologists play a crucial role in addressing conditions such as menstrual disorders, infertility, and menopause. They perform routine examinations, including Pap smears and pelvic exams, to ensure women's reproductive health.

II. **Obstetrician:** Obstetricians focus on pregnancy, childbirth, and postpartum care. They monitor the health of both the mother and the developing fetus, provide prenatal care, and assist with labor and delivery. Obstetricians manage high-risk pregnancies and address complications during childbirth. Their expertise ensures a safe and healthy pregnancy journey for women.

III. **Midwife:** Midwives specialize in providing personalized care and support during pregnancy, childbirth, and the postpartum period. They emphasize natural and holistic approaches to women's health, offering guidance on nutrition, childbirth education, and breastfeeding. Midwives often work in collaboration with obstetricians to ensure comprehensive care for expectant mothers.

IV. **Reproductive Endocrinologist:** Reproductive endocrinologists focus on addressing hormonal issues and infertility. They specialize in diagnosing and treating conditions that affect the endocrine system, impacting reproductive health. These specialists may offer fertility treatments, such as in vitro fertilization (IVF) and hormonal therapies, to assist individuals and couples in achieving pregnancy.

V. **Urogynecologist:** Urogynecologists specialize in the treatment of pelvic floor disorders, including urinary incontinence and pelvic organ prolapse. They address issues related to the muscles and connective tissues in the pelvic region. Urogynecologists may recommend surgical or non-surgical interventions to improve pelvic health and enhance the quality of life for women.

VI. **Women's Health Nurse Practitioner:** Women's health nurse practitioners are advanced practice nurses with specialized training in women's health. They provide a range of healthcare services, including routine exams, family planning, and preventive care. These practitioners often work collaboratively with physicians to deliver comprehensive and patient-centered care.

VII. **Breast Surgeon:** Breast surgeons specialize in the diagnosis and treatment of breast conditions, including breast cancer. They may perform breast biopsies, lumpectomies, mastectomies, and other surgical procedures. Breast surgeons work closely with oncologists and other specialists to create comprehensive treatment plans for breast health.

VIII. **Perinatologist (Maternal-Fetal Medicine Specialist):** Perinatologists, or maternal-fetal medicine specialists, focus on high-risk pregnancies. They provide specialized care for pregnant women with pre-existing medical conditions or complications that may affect the health of the mother or the developing fetus. Perinatologists collaborate with obstetricians to optimize outcomes for both mother and baby.

IX. **Pelvic Floor Physical Therapist:** Pelvic floor physical therapists specialize in addressing musculoskeletal issues related to the pelvic region. They provide non-invasive therapies to manage conditions such as pelvic pain, incontinence, and pelvic floor dysfunction. Pelvic floor physical therapy is often an integral part of comprehensive women's health care.

X. **Women's Health Psychologist:** Women's health psychologists focus on the psychological and emotional aspects of women's health. They address mental health issues such as anxiety, depression, and stress related to reproductive health, pregnancy, and menopause. These psychologists work in collaboration with other healthcare providers to ensure holistic care.

XI. **Endocrinologist:** Endocrinologists specialize in the endocrine system, which includes hormone-producing glands. In the context of women's health, endocrinologists play a crucial role in addressing hormonal imbalances that may affect reproductive health, menstrual cycles, and conditions such as polycystic ovary syndrome (PCOS) or thyroid disorders.

XII. **Genetic Counselor:** Genetic counselors specialize in assessing the risk of hereditary conditions and genetic disorders. In women's health, they may provide counseling for individuals or couples considering family planning, especially if there is a family history of genetic conditions. Genetic counselors offer information and support to make informed decisions about reproductive health.

XIII. **Dermatologist (Cosmetic Dermatology):** Dermatologists, particularly those specializing in cosmetic dermatology, address skin health concerns specific to women. This may include the management of skin conditions exacerbated by hormonal changes, such as acne during different life stages. Cosmetic dermatologists also provide aesthetic treatments to address skin aging.

XIV. **Nutritionist/Dietitian:** Nutritionists and dietitians specializing in women's health offer guidance on dietary choices that support hormonal balance, bone health, and overall well-being. They play a role in addressing conditions like obesity or eating disorders and provide nutritional advice during pregnancy and menopause.

XV. **Rheumatologist:** Rheumatologists specialize in autoimmune and inflammatory conditions that may disproportionately affect women, such as rheumatoid arthritis or lupus. These specialists work to manage symptoms, provide pain relief, and improve the quality of life for women dealing with these chronic conditions.

XVI. **Cardiologist:** Cardiologists focus on heart health, and in the context of women's health, they play a vital role in addressing cardiovascular conditions. Given that heart disease is a leading cause of death in women, cardiologists provide preventive care, diagnose heart-related issues, and develop treatment plans to protect heart health.

XVII. **Oncologist (Gynecologic Oncologist):** Gynecologic oncologists specialize in the diagnosis and treatment of cancers that affect the female reproductive system. This includes cancers of the ovaries, uterus, cervix, and other gynecologic organs. They collaborate with other specialists to provide comprehensive cancer care.

XVIII.   **Allergist/Immunologist:** Allergists and immunologists address allergic and immune system-related conditions that may impact women's health. This includes managing allergies, autoimmune disorders, and immunodeficiency conditions that can affect overall well-being.

XIX. **Neurologist:** Neurologists specializing in women's health may address neurological conditions that disproportionately affect women, such as migraines, multiple sclerosis, or neurological aspects of hormonal changes. They provide diagnosis, treatment, and management of neurological disorders.

XX. **Sleep Specialist:** Sleep specialists focus on addressing sleep-related issues that may impact women's health. Sleep disorders can have significant effects on overall well-being, hormonal balance, and mental health. Sleep specialists provide evaluations and treatments to improve sleep quality.

CONCLUSION

Recapitulation

1.   Support Systems and Resources during and after Menopause:

- Menopause is a natural phase in a woman's life, marked by the cessation of menstrual cycles and hormonal changes.
- Emotional support, lifestyle modifications, and medical interventions contribute to managing menopausal symptoms.
- Support systems encompass family, friends, healthcare providers, and online communities.
- Lifestyle changes include a balanced diet, regular exercise, and stress management.
- Cognitive Behavioral Therapy (CBT) offers psychological support during menopause.
- Hormone replacement therapy (HRT) and alternative therapies are medical interventions.

2.   Role of Hormones in Mental Health during Menopause:

- Hormonal fluctuations during menopause can impact mental health, leading to mood swings, anxiety, and depression.
- Estrogen plays a key role in neurotransmitter regulation, affecting mood and cognitive function.

- Hormone therapy and lifestyle changes are potential strategies to address mental health challenges.

3.   Cognitive Behavioral Therapy (CBT) for Menopausal Women:
- CBT is a therapeutic approach to address emotional and psychological challenges during menopause.
- It focuses on changing thought patterns and behaviors to improve mental well-being.
- CBT can help manage anxiety, depression, and stress associated with menopausal symptoms.

4.   Lifestyle Modifications during Menopause:
- Lifestyle changes include a balanced diet, regular exercise, and stress management.
- Adequate calcium and vitamin D intake support bone health during menopause.
- Limiting caffeine, alcohol, and quitting smoking contribute to overall well-being.

5.   Characteristics of Post-Menopause:
- Post-menopause follows menopause and is marked by the absence of menstrual cycles.
- Hormonal changes persist, impacting bone health, cardiovascular health, and overall well-being.

- Increased risk of osteoporosis and cardiovascular disease is associated with post-menopause.

6.   Embracing the Post-Menopausal Phase:
- Embracing post-menopause involves accepting and adapting to the changes in physical and emotional well-being.
- Lifestyle modifications, support systems, and self-care contribute to a positive post-menopausal experience.

7.   Persistence of Symptoms during Menopause:
- Some menopausal symptoms may persist into post-menopause.
- Symptom persistence requires ongoing management and support from healthcare providers.

8.   Importance of Ongoing Health Monitoring during Menopause:
- Regular health monitoring is crucial during menopause to address potential health risks.
- Screening for cardiovascular health, bone density, and mental well-being is essential.

9.   Support Systems and Resources during Menopause:

- Support systems encompass emotional support, healthcare providers, and community resources.
- Online communities and support groups provide a platform for sharing experiences and information.
- Professional guidance, lifestyle modifications, and alternative therapies contribute to holistic support.

10.   Lifestyle Changes for Heart Health in Post-Menopause:
- Post-menopausal women should adopt heart-healthy lifestyle changes.
- Regular exercise, a balanced diet, and stress management contribute to cardiovascular health.
- Monitoring cholesterol levels, blood pressure, and maintaining a healthy weight are crucial.

11.   Medications and Interventions for Cardiovascular Health during Post-Menopause:
- Medications and interventions may be prescribed to manage cardiovascular risks.
- Hormone therapy, statins, and lifestyle modifications are part of cardiovascular health management.

12.   Changes in Libido and Sexual Function during Post-Menopause:
- Hormonal changes and physical factors can impact libido and sexual function.

- Open communication with partners, addressing physical concerns, and seeking medical advice contribute to a healthy sexual life.

13.   Therapeutic Options for Sexual Health in Post-Menopause:
- Therapeutic options include hormonal treatments, lubricants, and lifestyle modifications.
- Open communication with healthcare providers and partners is essential for addressing sexual health.

14.   Acupuncture and Alternative Therapies in Integrative Women's Health:
- Acupuncture and alternative therapies offer holistic approaches to women's health.
- Acupuncture may address menstrual irregularities, menopausal symptoms, and fertility concerns.
- Herbal medicine complements acupuncture, providing remedies for menstrual and menopausal health.

15.   Support Groups and Communities for Resources in Women's Health:
- Support groups and communities are invaluable resources for emotional and informational support.

- They provide a sense of unity, shared experiences, and empowerment for women navigating health challenges.
- Online communities extend accessibility and inclusivity, fostering connections across diverse backgrounds.

16. Healthcare Providers and Specialists for Women's Health:
- Various healthcare providers play crucial roles in women's health, addressing diverse medical needs.
- Gynecologists, obstetricians, midwives, and specialists like endocrinologists and genetic counselors offer specialized care.
- Collaboration between healthcare professionals ensures comprehensive and personalized women's health care.

Empowering Women To Embrace Menopause And Post-Menopause

Menopause and the post-menopausal phase are transformative periods in a woman's life, marked by biological, psychological, and social changes. Rather than viewing this natural transition as a decline, it is crucial to empower women to embrace these phases with a positive mindset, fostering a sense of well-being and self-empowerment. This detailed exploration delves into the multifaceted aspects of empowering women during menopause and post-menopause, emphasizing a holistic approach that encompasses physical health, mental well-being, and societal perceptions.

I. **Shifting Perspectives:** Empowering women during menopause begins with a fundamental shift in perspectives. Instead of framing menopause as an end, it should be viewed as a new beginning—a stage of life that brings wisdom, experience, and an opportunity for self-discovery. Encouraging women to see this transition as a natural and empowering part of their journey is the first step.

II. **Comprehensive Education:** Knowledge is a powerful tool in empowerment. Providing comprehensive education about the physiological changes during menopause and post-menopause helps women understand what to expect. This includes information on hormonal shifts, bone health, cardiovascular changes, and the potential impact on mental well-being. Armed with knowledge, women can actively participate in managing their health.

III. **Holistic Self-Care Practices:** Empowering women involves nurturing the body, mind, and soul. Encouraging women to adopt holistic self-care practices, such as regular exercise, a balanced diet, and mindfulness techniques, contributes to overall well-being. Physical activities like yoga or tai chi can be particularly beneficial in promoting flexibility and reducing stress.

IV. **Redefining Beauty and Aging:** Societal perceptions of beauty often contribute to apprehensions about aging. Empowering women involves challenging and redefining these norms. Celebrating the beauty that comes with age, wisdom, and experience helps women embrace their changing bodies and appearance with confidence and self-assurance.

V. **Open Communication:** Creating an environment of open communication is essential. Women should feel encouraged to discuss their experiences, concerns, and emotions related to menopause without judgment. Supportive networks, whether comprised of friends, family, or healthcare professionals, play a crucial role in fostering a sense of understanding and validation.

VI. **Mental Health Support:** Menopause can impact mental health, leading to mood swings, anxiety, or depression. Empowering women involves acknowledging and addressing these mental health aspects. Offering support services, such as counseling or support groups, provides a safe space for women to express their emotions and navigate the psychological aspects of this life stage.

VII. **Embracing Sexual Health:** Empowering women during menopause involves recognizing and addressing changes in sexual health. Open conversations with healthcare providers about concerns or challenges can lead to solutions, ensuring that women feel confident and empowered in their sexual well-being during and after menopause.

VIII. **Encouraging Pursuit of Passions:** Menopause often coincides with a time when many women have more personal freedom. Encouraging them to pursue passions, hobbies, or career aspirations can be empowering. This phase offers an opportunity for self-discovery and personal growth, reinforcing the idea that life is rich and fulfilling beyond the reproductive years.

IX. **Fostering Independence:** Independence is a key element of empowerment. Encouraging women to take charge of their health, make informed decisions, and actively participate in their healthcare journey fosters a sense of independence. This can include being proactive in seeking medical advice, making lifestyle choices, and advocating for their well-being.

X. **Community and Peer Support:** Empowerment is amplified in a supportive community. Facilitating connections with peers who are navigating similar experiences creates a sense of solidarity. Women's health support groups, both online and offline, provide a platform for sharing insights, advice, and encouragement, reinforcing the idea that women are not alone in their journey.

XI. **Reinforcing Positive Aging Narratives:** Society often perpetuates negative stereotypes about aging. Empowering women involves challenging and reshaping these narratives. Highlighting positive stories of women thriving in their post-menopausal years showcases the diversity and strength that comes with age, inspiring others to embrace this phase with optimism.

XII. **Personalized Healthcare Strategies:** Acknowledging that each woman's experience with menopause is unique, empowering women involves tailoring healthcare strategies to individual needs. Personalized approaches, whether in hormone therapy, nutrition plans, or mental health support, contribute to a sense of agency and control over one's well-being.

XIII. **Emphasizing Life Beyond Reproduction:** Empowering women during and after menopause involves emphasizing that life holds abundant possibilities beyond the reproductive years. Women can redirect their focus towards personal goals, career aspirations, or educational pursuits, recognizing that their value extends far beyond traditional societal expectations.

XIV. **Advocacy for Women's Health:** Empowerment on an individual level can translate into broader advocacy efforts. Encouraging women to be advocates for women's health, challenging societal norms, and participating in conversations that destigmatize menopause contribute to a collective empowerment that transcends individual experiences.

www.ingramcontent.com/pod-product-compliance
Lightning Source LLC
Chambersburg PA
CBHW070922260726
48661CB00003B/794